Coping with Medications

Coping with Aging Series

Series Editor
John C. Rosenbek, Ph.D.
Chief, Speech Pathology and Audiology Services
William S. Middleton Memorial Hospital
Madison, Wisconsin

Medical Editor
Molly Carnes, M.D.
Department of Medicine and Institute on Aging
University of Wisconsin
Madison, Wisconsin

Chief, Geriatrics Section
William S. Middleton Memorial Hospital
Madison, Wisconsin

Published in Cooperation with
the National Council of Senior Citizens

Coping with Medications

Maren E. Meyer, FASCP
Pharmacist

SINGULAR PUBLISHING GROUP, INC.
SAN DIEGO, CALIFORNIA

Illustrations by
Jane Huff Linderud

Published by Singular Publishing Group, Inc.
4284 41st Street
San Diego, California 92105-1197

© **1993 by Singular Publishing Group, Inc.**

Typeset in 11/14 Times by CFW Graphics
Printed in the United States of America by McNaughton & Gunn

Library of Congress Cataloging-in-Publication Data

Meyer, Maren E.
    Coping with medications / Maren E. Meyer.
      p.   cm. — (Coping with aging series)
    Includes bibliographical references.
    ISBN 1-879105-67-5
    1. Geriatric pharmacology—Popular works. 2. Aged—Drug use—
—Safety measures. 3. Aged — Life skills guides. I. Title.
II. Series.
RC953.7.M48   1992
615.5′80846—dc20

92-25613
CIP

❖ Table of Contents

❖ Foreword

The books in the *Coping with Aging Series* are written for men and women coping with the challenges of aging, and for their families and other caregivers. The authors are all experienced practitioners: doctors, nurses, social workers, psychologists, pharmacists, nutritionists, audiologists, physical and occupational therapists, and speech-language pathologists.

The topics of individual volumes are as varied as are the challenges that aging may bring. These include: hearing loss, low vision, depression, sexual dysfunction, immobility, intellectual impairment, language impairment, speech impairment, swallowing impairment, death and dying, bowel and bladder incontinence, stress of caregiving, giving up independence, medications, and stroke. The volumes themselves, however, share common features. Foremost, they are practical, jargon-free, and responsible. Each contains professionally valid information translated into language people who are not health care providers can understand. Each contains useful advice and sections to help readers decide how they are doing and whether they need to do more, do less, or do something different. Each includes lists of services, suppliers, and additional readings. Each provides evidence that no single person need cope alone.

None of the volumes can substitute for appropriate professional health care. However, when combined with the care, instruction, and counseling that health care providers supply, they make coping with aging easier.

America is greying at the same time its treasury is inadequate to meet its population's needs. Thus the *Coping with Aging Series* offers help for people who need and want to help themselves.

This volume, *Coping with Medications,* is written by a professional clinical pharmacist with over 10 years of experience working with people who take medications. She has designed this book to be a source of information to make you a more informed consumer of medications, and she offers practical suggestions to assist you in managing your medications. If you, or someone you know, is having difficulty figuring out your medications, this book may help. If you want to know more about how your medications work, what the names of your medications mean, what questions to ask your doctor, how to keep track of your medications, the most efficient way to get your prescriptions filled, how to watch for side effects of your medications, or how to travel with your medications, this book will give you answers in words you can understand.

John C. Rosenbek, Ph.D.
Series Editor

Molly Carnes, M.D.
Medical Editor

❖ Preface

The goal and purpose of *Coping With Medications* is to help you and your loved ones be as safe, independent, and effective in the management of medications as possible. It is intended to help you develop sufficient understanding about your medications to live with them comfortably. In preparing this book, I discovered some interesting theories on aging, the aging memory, and the ability to learn new things.

One developmental theory can be summarized in this way. The young human mind is like a new and empty filing cabinet. Information gets tucked into the drawers "willy-nilly." As time goes by, the mind begins sorting the information, deciding what bits belong together. It creates files of information. In the elderly human mind, the file cabinet drawers are packed with files and loose bits of information. When the older mind is presented with new information, it seems to take a longer period of time processing the new data. It's not necessarily that the older mind can't store the new information, perhaps it's that the older mind wants to file it in the correct place and has more files to choose from. I mention this as a reminder to the reader that not all theories view aging in terms of decline.

The fact is that, like many things we do, medication-taking behaviors are not born to us. We have to learn them. Generally, unless we have had childhood or young adult chronic diseases, we don't develop these skills until we are older adults. As we age, we seem to accumulate more and more chronic conditions that are treated with medication. While we have probably been exposed to medication administration and management when we gave our children antibiotics for ear infections, for example, *we* probably never had to take medications daily "for the rest of our lives." Medication management is just another of the many skills that people learn as they live and age.

I want you to become a great problem solver. There is a natural order in tracking down exactly what a problem is all about. Learning a logical sequence for solving problems will help you identify the issues, determine what the obstacles are and how they can best be overcome. It is valuable to learn which health professionals are the best information sources for various types of problems. One of our toughest decisions is determining where compromise is possible or acceptable. With all this in mind, we can set a time frame for making changes. Naturally, we will evaluate and reevaluate our progress and changing needs. The beauty of a sound systematic approach is that the skills will apply even when the nature of the problem is altered.

Finally, a cautionary note. The more we learn the more we should realize how little we really know and understand. The body of information that is called health care is tremendously vast and, in order to cope with it, we will be relying on experts in many areas. Poorly applied, misunderstood, or outdated information can be as dangerous as an absence of knowledge. Friends, publications, and the media provide an ongoing source of good and poor information. Updating our ideas and habits is a challenge. As technological changes occur, the methods we have traditionally used to help us stay healthy are under fire. Fortunately, you have the members of *your* health care team to help you make decisions that will be safe and satisfying to you.

❖ Acknowledgments

Special thanks go to the following people for their help in preparing this book: Ed Rahn, Pharmacist; Howard Backe, Pharmacist; Joe Mastalski, Pharmacist; Joan Berndt; Caregiver; Ruth Krueger, Teacher; and Stephanie Cerny, Child and Family Studies.

Chapter 1

America's Other Drug Problem

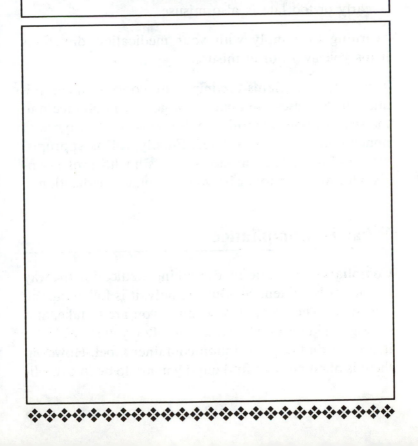

America's "other drug problem" is not one of street criminals or rebellious youth, it is the misuse of legitimate medications. The dangers from this misuse are as well established as the other kinds of drug problems.

1. When a drug is used for a rational therapeutic reason, it is being used as a medication.

2. Taking a drug for any other reason is misuse.

3. The inappropriate use of your own medications or taking someone else's medication is misuse.

4. Taking too many or too few doses or taking them too early or too late is also misuse.

Learning to comply with your medication directions helps you avoid drug misuse.

This chapter explains the important concept of compliance. It discusses the benefits of good compliance and the risks of poor compliance. Reasons for and types of noncompliance are described. Finally, it lists appropriate uses for medication and suggests health professionals who are able to assist you with your medication.

What is Compliance

Compliance can be defined as taking medication the way the prescriber intended. Quite simply, it is following the directions. The dose, or how much you are to take, and dosing schedule, or when and how often you should take it, appear on the prescription container label. However, there is often more to find out if you are to be in compliance. It is important for you to know exactly what the prescriber has in mind regarding the medication therapy. You need to know:

1. How long the medication must be taken.

2. If the medication should be taken regularly or only when you have symptoms.

3. How often to check with your doctor about your progress on the medication.

4. What to do if you are concerned about the medication's action or side effects.

The whole health care team wants you to be healthy and knows that your therapy is not likely to succeed without your participation, understanding, and compliance. They will do all they can, but finally, medication compliance becomes a personal responsibility.

Advantages of Compliance

Here are five important reasons for complying with instructions.

1. *Getting the desired outcome of therapy.* This could mean achieving stable blood sugar if you have diabetes or stabilizing blood pressure if you have hypertension, curing an infection, having a rash go away or getting pain under control.

2. *Reducing the risk of a recurrence of the same condition.* For example, the bacteria that cause an infection may not be entirely eliminated if you fail to finish the course of

therapy. Unless you finish the antibiotic as directed there is an increased risk that the bacteria may grow back and cause illness again.

3. *Lowering the risk of consequences from the disease being treated.* For example, good blood pressure control reduces the risk of having a stroke.

4. *Decreasing the risk of unwanted side effects from your medication.* For example, when medication intended to be taken with food is taken on an empty stomach, discomfort may result. This situation could be avoided by good compliance with directions.

5. *Knowing that you have done everything you can do to successfully treat your condition.* With an irreversible or progressive condition, it is important for you and the people who care about you to realize that you are doing everything possible to optimize your well being.

Most people want to be as healthy as they possibly can be. They want the advantages of good compliance and want to avoid the risks of noncompliance. So why is it that people sometimes don't comply despite the risks? This question has been studied extensively. Before answering it, however, let's consider the risks of noncompliance.

Risks of Medication Noncompliance

Medication noncompliance can cause the following:

1. *Noncompliance can lead to adverse drug reactions.* An example is taking bisacodyl tablets, a common laxative, with food. This results in the medication dissolving too

soon in the intestinal tract and leads to unpleasant stomach pains.

2. *Noncompliance can lead to preventable hospitalizations.* In fact, it has been shown that these hospitalizations could be reduced by as much as 29 percent in older adults if medications are used properly (Col et al., 1990).

3. *Noncompliance means the health condition for which the medicine was prescribed goes untreated or is poorly treated.* This can occur from use of outdated medication that may not be potent enough to treat the condition effectively. This problem also occurs when the medication is taken in doses less than the one prescribed.

4. *Noncompliance can increase suffering and the cost of therapy.* Suppose a person is prescribed an antibiotic for a sinus infection with directions to take one capsule three times daily for 14 days. If the person fails to comply with the directions, stopping the medication after 7 days, the condition might persist. In a case such as this, the condition may have to be reassessed by the physician, and a different antibiotic might be required. This means noncompliance causes the person to suffer longer than he or she would have if therapy had been correctly completed. Furthermore, an extra doctor's visit and possibly a second prescription would be required.

5. *Noncompliance makes it impossible to determine what changes in therapy might improve the outcome.* The prescriber may adjust the dose based on incorrect information. For example, a person has been prescribed theophylline tablets to be taken three times daily to improve breathing. The person complains that his or her breath-

ing is still difficult and uncomfortable. This person fails to tell the doctor that only two pills are being taken daily instead of the prescribed three. The prescriber may believe the medication would give better results if the patient took a higher dose such as four tablets daily. In fact, the person would get a higher dose by just taking the medication three times daily as first prescribed. To compound the problem, if the person does decide to take four tablets daily, he or she may suffer serious side effects.

6. *Noncompliance in the form of inconsistent medication use may lead to a high rate of side effects.* For example, randomly starting and stopping medications taken for depression can lead to a higher than usual incidence of side effects. These and numerous other medications typically have side effects that become less problematic with regular use. Generally, people develop a tolerance to the drowsiness associated with some anti-depressants in a week or 10 days. Stopping the medication can cause this tolerance to be lost. When a person starts and stops medications, he or she may be constantly confronted with side effects that would otherwise be experienced during only the initial phase of therapy.

Types of Noncompliance

There are two main types of noncompliance — intentional and unintentional. It is useful for the health care team to know why a particular person does not comply with the medication regimen. By identifying the reason, the team can help to eliminate it.

After explaining what is meant by each type of noncompliance, some statements are included that may be heard from people who fall into each category.

Intentional Noncompliance

Intentional noncompliance occurs as the result of a conscious decision not to follow the directions. Intentional noncompliance seems to arise when people have unasked or unanswered questions and concerns about a medication. These questions can result from lack of information or from inaccurate ideas. Usually, intentional noncompliance involves a one-sided decision by a person without discussion with members of the health care team.

Statements like the following often indicate that a person is intentionally not complying.

"I feel better so I'm not taking it anymore."

"I didn't think that medication was helping, so I quit taking it."

"I take it when I have symptoms but not all the time."

"I'm trying to save some money so I cut out a dose."

"I started having side effects that I know were caused by the drug."

Unintentional Noncompliance

Unintentional noncompliance is the result of an error or misunderstanding. The patient is often not aware that the way he or she is taking the medicine is not how the prescriber intended it to be taken. Statements like those following may indicate unintentional, but significant, noncompliance.

"I thought the doctor told me to take only one tablet a day."

"I can't read the labels."

"I was sure the doctor told me to quit taking that medication."

"This looked like my medication, but it turns out that it is my husband's."

"I just plain forget."

Obstacles to Good Compliance

The National Council on Patient Information and Education consists of more than 260 member organizations representing health care including consumer groups, manufacturers, and government agencies. Its sole goal is to promote the safe and effective use of medications. The Council describes some of the most common obstacles to compliance as:

1. *The longer the therapy lasts, the more medication compliance drops.* Thus, the person who is facing a 7-day course of antibiotics may be more apt to complete the therapy *as directed* than a person faced with taking medication daily for the rest of his or her life.

2. *As the number of medications a person must take increases, noncompliance becomes a bigger problem.* It's one

thing to remember to take one pill twice a day, but remembering to have three pills on hand to take twice a day is tougher. It's like the difference between juggling one item and juggling three.

3. *The greater the number of daily doses people must take, the worse their compliance.* Some people have to remember to take doses six or eight times daily. This means they have to devote a lot of time and thought to remembering when a dose is needed and what medication it should be.

4. *When medication schedules aren't adapted to patient lifestyles, compliance suffers.* Some heart medications must be taken around the clock. Most people, however, are reluctant to get up in the middle of the night to take medication. Sustained release forms of many of these medications are now available. Fortunately, your pharmacist and prescriber can usually find these and other alternatives that fit your lifestyle and make compliance easier.

5. *Some people forget to take medication.* Compliance can be significantly improved by writing down instructions. Having the written directions posted prominently helps people remember.

Compliance is more difficult if a person is unable to see and to read. It is estimated that 20 percent of all adults cannot read (Kaestle and Damon-Moore, 1991). In addition, many older adults have problems with vision (Kosnik et al., 1988). People who for whatever reason cannot read need to be identified so instructions can be provided in a more useful way. People who are unable to read will need to memorize their medications including when and how to take them. Other instructional aids may be helpful to those with low vision. For example, directions can be written in large bold print, or universal symbols can be used to tell the information. Tear-off calendars and medication organizers are other options. These aids are described in Chapter 18.

6. *When physicians, nurses, or pharmacists don't have time to spend with patients, compliance may diminish, especially for older people.* Compliance isn't easy and most people need reinforcement and teaching. Ongoing communication and feedback from the health care team promotes compliance.

The Right Not to Comply

As part of the health care team, each person shares responsibility for the outcome of medication therapy. People have the right and the responsibility to ask questions and learn the pros and cons of either taking or omitting a medication from their therapy. They have the right to refuse therapy. Exercising that right, however, should be an informed decision involving the rest of the health care team.

In summary, always take medication as directed by the prescriber. If you have problems with side effects, the dose, or schedule, inform the prescriber. If problems occur, it is generally possible to find an alternative approach. Good communication with your health care team will go a long way toward helping your medications succeed for you. It will also help you avoid becoming part of America's "other drug problem."

Chapter 2

The Health Care Team

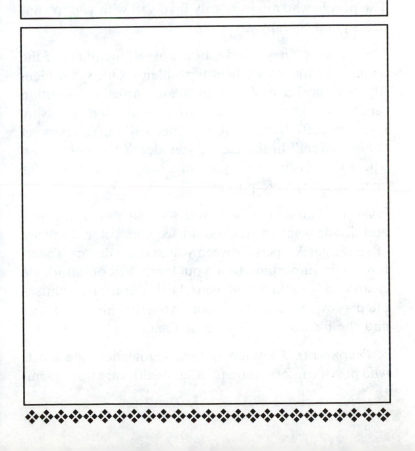

The concept of a health care team is relatively new. This chapter describes possible members of your health care team and how they can help you get the most from your medications. There are probably more health care professionals involved in your medication care than you suppose. Keep in mind, the most indispensable member of the team is you and without your cooperation the team cannot help.

Your Primary Team

The people who are primarily involved with you in your medication therapy are:

1. *Physicians.* They are the best trained members of the team to diagnose your health problems. Once they identify your health problem, they may order prescription medication and any follow-up tests needed to assure safety and effectiveness of your medication. You may get the best overall health care if you identify one physician who will coordinate all your medical care and serve as your "primary care physician."

2. *Nurses.* Nurses can help you sort out your symptoms and decide whether you should see the doctor. They are often the gatekeepers between you and the doctor. Therefore, it is important that you learn to communicate clearly with them about your health concerns. Nurses often provide education about your health conditions and the methods used to treat them.

3. *Pharmacists.* They are trained medication specialists who provide information to other health care team mem-

bers and to you. Pharmacists dispense the medications and associated products ordered by your doctor and give the counseling that contributes to the medications' safety and effectiveness. Pharmacists can help you devise methods to improve your compliance. They keep records of your prescription medications and can help you choose nonprescription medication wisely.

4. *Social Workers.* They can help you resolve problems that may be keeping you from getting good health care. These problems may be anything from finances to transportation to family disapproval or interference. Many social workers have experience and an interest in helping you comply with your medication regimen.

The Secondary Team

Other health care professionals who can influence your medication and medication-taking behavior include:

1. *Dieticians.* Besides helping you to maintain a healthy diet for normal living, they can help you identify specific dietary needs that may help to control a disease you have. They are a good source of information about how food interacts with your medications.

2. *Occupational Therapists.* They can help you with the general management of your household, offer suggestions and provide devices that may make medication compliance easier for you. They often are involved in helping institutionalized people learn about and gain control of their medication regimens before being discharged.

3. *Physical Therapists.* They help you maintain and improve your strength and mobility. These assets help you remain independent and able to attain a lifestyle in which you can manage your everyday affairs including your medications.

4. *Dentists.* They can help you detect problems related to the impact of medicines on your mouth. It is important not to neglect symptoms like dry mouth caused by many medications. In addition, dentists can help you remain well nourished by assuring that your dentures fit well and your teeth and gums are in good health.

5. *Eye Care Specialists.* By helping you get the optimal eyeglass prescription, they can directly affect your ability to read medication labels. These professionals can also help you treat the drying effects that some medication has on your eyes.

6. *Podiatrists.* They can help you take good care of your feet even though you may not be able to bend enough to do this yourself. Because the condition of your feet can reveal a great deal about the quality of disease control in such diseases as diabetes, foot care is an important monitor of overall health care.

7. *Physician Specialists.* This group of practitioners includes ophthalmologists, urologists, cardiologists, rheumatologists, neurologists, psychiatrists, and many others. These doctors may become more involved as a health condition worsens. Ultimately, they should work closely with your primary care physician regarding medication prescribing. As the number of physicians caring for your health increases, the importance of having a personal

pharmacist grows. Your pharmacist can provide information to both your primary care physician and to the specialist, thus avoiding duplications in medication therapy and drug interactions.

8. *Speech Pathologists.* They can help determine whether you have a swallowing problem. They can recommend changes in the consistency of foods and beverages you consume with your medications.

9. *Audiologists.* These specialists can help you hear as well as possible so you can get the full benefit from your interactions with the rest of the health care team.

Other People Who Can Help With Your Medications

In addition to the health care professionals just discussed, the following people can also assist you.

1. *Representatives of Your Religion.* If your religion opposes the use of medications, it is particularly important for you to come to a working arrangement with your church and the health care team. When your illness is severe, it is especially comforting to have the support of members of your religion. In addition, fellow church members are often among the most reliable helpers you will find.

2. *Pharmacy Assistants.* These team members can help you with your insurance claims, questions about product availability, and deliveries. Their familiarity with you works in your favor when health matters don't go well.

3. *Your Family and/or Caregiver.* These people are rooting for your success. They are probably not the best sources of medication information, but they can help you solve health care problems and stay organized. They are especially helpful when they encourage you to stick to your medication regimen.

Of course, not all health care teams have all these members, but it is possible. When you need a service or some sound advice about your health care, contact one or more of these people.

Chapter 3

How Do Medications Work?

Pharmacology is the study of the way medications work. What we know about pharmacology affects what medications are prescribed for you and how they are to be taken. This chapter will introduce you to pharmacology and give you an idea of what happens when you take medication. Fortunately, pharmacology is divided into several easily understood segments. The information in these segments explains many of the questions you might have about your medication.

Components of Pharmacology

Once a dose of medication is prescribed, there are six main issues to consider in getting the desired results from medication.

1. How the medication gets into the body

2. How the medication is dissolved and absorbed into the body

3. Distribution of the medication to the different areas within the body

4. Action of the medication on the tissues

5. Metabolism or breakdown of the medication

6. Elimination of the medication and its breakdown products from the body.

Each of the issues above deals with a part of the process of getting the desired results from medication. By examining these individually, you will get a clearer picture of why things happen the way they do with medications.

Getting the Medication Into Your Body

Medications can get into the body by several routes. In this section, each route of administering medication is described with examples and special considerations.

By Mouth

The most common way to take medication is by mouth or orally. The dose may take the form of pills, tablets, capsules, or oral liquids. An oral dose is swallowed, travels down the esophagus and into the stomach.

Nasal Inhalation

Some medication is administered by inhaling it through the nose. In this case, the medication as an aerosolized liquid or fine powder is sprayed and absorbed into the moist lining of the nasal passages. The most commonly used nasal sprays contain solutions or suspensions of decongestants, steroids, or salt/saline. These products are frequently used to moisten dry nasal membranes or treat congested inflamed nasal passages. The advantage of this route of administration is that the medication generally stays in the nasal passages and doesn't affect the rest of your body.

Oral Inhalation

Similarly, there are medications that are taken by oral inhalation. The inhalers or "puffers" used by asthmatics are in this group. A fine mist of liquid or powdered medication is inhaled through the mouth. Often the medication is delivered from a pressurized container.

The intention with these products is that the medication is delivered into the lower part of the lungs.

Injection

Other medications can only be given by injection, either (a) subcutaneously, (b) intramuscularly, or (c) intravenously.

Subcutaneous administration is the delivery of a medication right under the skin. It is used in most insulin administration.

Intramuscular means into the muscle. The muscles used most in this method are the gluteus maximus (buttocks) and the deltoid (upper arm). Some vaccines, pain medications, and antibiotics are given by intramuscular injection.

The intravenous route delivers medication directly into the bloodstream. Antibiotics, pain medications, and cancer chemotherapy drugs are the medicines most often given by this method. This method was once used almost exclusively in the hospital setting. Now, however, people may receive some intravenous medications at home or in their doctors' offices.

Injection is used for delivering medications that would be broken down by stomach acid or that are poorly absorbed through the intestinal tract. Injection is also used to speed the administration and effects from medication in critical situations. In the emergency room, many medications are administered by injection. When medication is injected, it is usually delivered quickly and efficiently to body tissues. Special training should be expected of any person using injectable medications. This is because the risk from errors is even greater than if the medication is administered by some other route.

Vaginal and Rectal

Vaginal and rectal routes are used to administer some medications. Vaginal administration is appropriate when the vagina is the tissue being treated. Treatment of vaginal yeast infection is an example. Vaginal medications are available as suppositories, creams, and douches.

Drugs given by rectal suppositories or enemas are inserted into the rectum. This route may by used to treat the bowel as in the treatment of inflammatory bowel diseases. Other rectal preparations may be absorbed to treat conditions in the rest of the body. For example, some pain medications are available as rectal suppositories. When patients are unable to take oral medications, as in patients who have severe nausea and vomiting, rectal administration might be favored.

Topical

Topical application of medication means applying it to the skin or mucous membranes. Medications *absorbed through* the skin or the lining of the mouth are intended to act elsewhere in the body. Both nitroglycerin topical ointment and nitroglycerin sublingual (under the tongue) tablets are in this category.

Some medications are applied to the skin to treat skin conditions. It is *not intended* that these preparations be absorbed into the body. Such medications include ear and eye drops and topical creams, ointments, and gels for rashes and other skin conditions.

Dissolution and Absorption

Regardless of how they are administered, medications must get absorbed before they can act. The step that determines the rate at which a medication gets absorbed is its dissolution. *Dissolution* is how fast and completely a medication dissolves. To be absorbed, a medication must be dissolved. Only then can it cross cell barriers. It is important for medication to dissolve reliably and consistently. This assures you that each time you take the medication the onset of action will be about the same. It also means that about the same amount or dose of medication will be available to get to tissues and act. Medications are engineered to offer the same expected dose each time they are taken.

Here are some problems that can impede dissolution of medications and/or cause slow absorption.

1. *Medication can be slowed as it passes through the esophagus to the stomach by taking it with too little liquid.* In this case, dissolution will be slow. This is one reason your pharmacist may add a label to remind you to take medicine with plenty of water.

2. *Stomach acid can break down or inactivate some medications as they dissolve.* Insulin is an example. It will not work if given by mouth; it must be given by injection. Sublingual nitroglycerin is another example of medicine that is broken down by stomach acid. It is administered by allowing the active ingredient to be absorbed through the lining of the mouth or through the skin.

3. *Other medications require stomach acid in order to work.* The anti-ulcer medication sucralfate (i.e., Carafate, a

registered trademark of Marion Merrill Dow, Inc.) dissolves and works best in acidic conditions. This generally means in an empty stomach.

4. *Some medications are only absorbed in a specific part of the intestines.* Iron supplements, for example, are mainly absorbed in one part of the intestinal tract. Because of this, time-released iron preparations may be less completely absorbed than regular iron tablets.

It is important to remember that when dissolution of an oral medication is slowed, the absorption will be affected. This can alter the onset of medication action, the extent that the medication is present in the blood, and the effectiveness of the medication.

Distribution to the Tissues

Blood is responsible for transporting most medications to the different tissues of the body. Many medications attach themselves to proteins in the blood. Some important drug interactions occur when medications compete for transport sites on these proteins. While medications are attached to proteins in the blood they cannot enter the tissues and so are not able to exert their usual action. To use a sports' analogy, these medications could be viewed as sitting out the game on the bench. For a medication to work, it must let go of the protein. Once free in the bloodstream, it is able to travel to the tissues where it can act. This is akin to it being off the bench and in the game. The amount of medication available to enter the tissues and exhibit its action can be greatly influenced by anything that affects its attachment to proteins in the blood. Once they are in the bloodstream, medications are delivered to both healthy and ill tissues.

Ideally, to minimize unwanted side effects, medication would be delivered only to the site or tissue where it is needed. Advances in medication delivery systems have made this possible in some cases. An example of specific medication delivery is the use of a nasal decongestant spray. It treats only the nasal passages. Taking an oral decongestant will clear up nasal congestion, but it unnecessarily exposes most of your body cells to the medication. Another example is the delivery of cancer chemotherapy medications to their specific sites of action. In this way, only the cancer cells are killed while the healthy cells and tissues are maintained. Biotechnology and the new delivery systems are creating ways to treat only the specific tissues involved in an illness.

Action on the Cells and Tissues

If an adequate amount of medication has been absorbed and distributed to the tissues, the medication's effect can occur. Depending on the nature of the medication itself, the effect may be immediate or delayed. A medication like epinephrine, given by injection in an emergency, acts immediately. Injectable medications for surgical anesthesia also act immediately. Some medications must reach a particular level or concentration in the blood before results are evident. An example is medication for depression, where days or weeks can pass before an effect is noted. It is useful to know this information so you are aware of how quickly your medication will work.

The actual mechanism by which a medication acts varies. For most products, it is not too well understood. We do know that each medication can act at many locations. The resulting actions give us the desired effect along with side effects. Muscle relaxants, for example, act both at skeletal muscle, which is their intended site of action, and in the brain to cause drowsiness as a side effect.

Metabolism or Breakdown of the Medication

One way your body keeps medications from building up is by inactivating them. When medications are released from the sites of their activity, they are carried in the blood to the liver where many medications are broken down or metabolized. If your liver does not function well in breaking down a medication, the effects of the medication might last much longer than desired. In this case, each extra dose taken might bring you closer to toxic levels of the medication. As long as medications are broken down to inactive products, their effects on tissues end. To maintain the medication's activity in your body, you have to take medication often enough to replace what is being broken down. Depending on the characteristics of the medication and your body's ability to break it down, you may have to take medication one to six times a day.

Elimination of Medications and Breakdown Products

Our best system for getting rid of medications and their breakdown products in the blood is through the urine. Your kidneys filter out the waste in your bloodstream and concentrate it in your urine. Urine is removed from the body by urination. If kidney function is inadequate, waste products from routine cell activities along with medications may build up in your body. This situation can be the result of an illness such as diabetes. When kidney impairment is severe, dialysis may be used to keep the blood in proper balance and to keep medication from building up in the body.

Your health care team monitors your kidney function with laboratory tests. Because kidney function declines with age, the dosage of many medications is reduced for elderly patients.

Applications of Pharmacology

This is all interesting enough, but what practical applications does it have for you as a patient or caregiver?

1. If you take oral medications without adequate liquids you may slow the rate at which the medication dissolves. This can slow the onset of action of the medication.

2. Taking a handful of medications all at one time can also cause problems with dissolution. Think about how differently large and small lumps of flour or cocoa dis-

solve. You get quicker more reliable dissolution by taking the pills one at a time with water in between.

3. If you are extremely thin, doctors may hesitate to give you intramuscular injections. Very thin patients may not have adequate blood flow to the injection site to get the medication absorbed and into circulation. This could lead to the medical condition being inadequately treated.

4. Areas with poor blood flow or blood pooling such as diabetic foot ulcers and abscesses may not receive enough medication from the blood stream to be immediately helpful. These conditions often require prolonged intensive therapy.

5. If you are very poorly nourished, you may have reduced proteins in your blood. Medications that are carried on these proteins then have a greater amount of the medication floating free in the blood. This portion of the medication is free to act on tissues while the portion bound to proteins is not. This situation could result in a greater response than expected from a low medication dosage.

6. A person with decreased heart strength will pump less blood to the liver. Because most medications get broken down and inactivated by the liver, medications may last longer in the body in such a person. The medication dosage or dosing schedule would have to be adjusted to keep the active medication from building up.

7. Taking medication while reclining can cause it to lodge in your esophagus. This could cause discomfort and slow the dissolution time. The medication would not

begin to act as quickly as it should. Esophageal irritation could also occur.

This introduction to pharmacology may help you as you learn more about your medications. The more informed you are about all aspects of medication the safer you'll be when you handle it. The more you learn, the more you understand why and how to comply with your medication regimen.

Chapter 4

Medication Allergies

It is important to recognize and alert your health care team to any medication allergies you may have. This chapter describes medication allergies and how they differ from other adverse reactions to medications. Adverse reactions are also called side effects.

Allergic Reactions

In an allergic reaction, your body views a medication you've taken as a harmful foreign substance. There are different types of allergic reactions to medications. Some begin almost immediately after you take a medication while others may begin only after days of exposure to the medication. An allergic reaction may occur when cells in your immune system mount an attack against the medication you have taken. When this happens, many cells in your immune system release chemicals in an attempt to destroy the medication they view as a foreign substance. These chemicals are responsible for the symptoms seen in allergic reactions. There may be a rash, swelling, shortness of breath, and even shock. An allergic reaction to a medication can be a minor annoyance or a medical emergency.

With a true medication allergy, a reaction will probably occur every time you are exposed to the offending substance. You may also have an allergic reaction to other medications that are chemically similar to the one to which you are allergic. For example, if you have a penicillin allergy, some antibiotics in a group of medications called cephalosporins may also cause you problems.

Be sure to let your doctor or pharmacist know about any allergies you have to medications. Remember that allergies are not limited to just prescription medicines. Over the counter (OTC) medications can also cause allergies.

Adverse Reactions

Much of what people regard as allergies are actually side effects or adverse drug reactions or they may be medication intolerance. The distinction between adverse reactions and allergic reactions is *very* important. Being incorrectly labeled as allergic to a medication might keep you from being successfully treated with that medication because of fear of an allergic reaction. Since there are occasions when a particular medicine may save your life, it is a good idea to find out whether you truly have an allergy to it.

Besides having the effects you want, *all* medications have some other effects. You may or may not desire these side effects. You may or may not experience them. If they are unpleasant or undesirable, they are called adverse reactions. Adverse effects (or reactions) can be as simple as causing a bad taste in your mouth or as severe as causing damage to your kidneys.

Here's an example. Diphenhydramine is an OTC medication used to treat coughing, allergies, and insomnia. Some of these beneficial effects are actually a result of its side effects. For instance, the sedation it causes is one of its side effects. This permits the medication to be used therapeutically in nonprescription sleep aids for insomnia. Though these products are marketed under different brand names, the chemical in them is diphenhydramine. If the sedation is not desired and is experienced when taking diphenhydramine for some other reason, you'd call the sedation an adverse effect.

Another case is that of codeine. Codeine is a narcotic. It has properties for cough suppression, pain relief, and drowsiness. The latter is a side effect and can be useful when pain keeps you awake. Another side effect of codeine is nausea and vomiting. This occurs at different doses for different people. If it occurs at a dose used for pain, it is undesirable and thus is an adverse effect.

You might want the medication record kept by your doctor and pharmacist to show that you don't want to get a particular medication because of adverse effects you have experienced.

Adverse effects are an expected result of the chemical action of a medication. Allergies are not. It is difficult to predict how many people will develop an allergy to a medication, but we know the degree of risk for adverse effects. It will often take an expert to determine the difference. A safe approach is to keep good records of the medications you take and of reactions that might occur while you are taking them. You and your physician and pharmacist can work together to determine which medications are safe for you to use.

Chapter 5

Learning About Your Medications

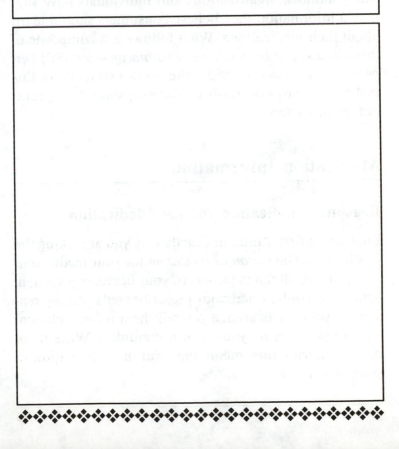

Medications are not simple, but by using a structured plan you can learn a lot about them. The secret is to start simply, build a solid foundation, and add at your own pace. By approaching the topic systematically, you will be able to assess the benefits and risks of various medications. Before you can master all the information suggested below, you will be taking the medication. Each time you prepare to take a dose, glance again at the directions on the prescription vial. The information that follows is intended to supplement, not replace, the label directions.

Many authors, organizations and individuals have suggested information they believe consumers should learn about their medications. What follows is a composite of these items. The *United States Pharmacopoeia* (USP) *Dispensing Information* provides the overall structure of this system and forms the basis for the worksheet that accompanies this chapter.

Medication Information

Reason or Indication for the Medication

First things first. Find out exactly why you are taking the medication. The *reason or indication* for your medication tells you and all the members of your health team much. Almost certainly, when your prescriber tells you the reason for your medications, you will hear a few technical words that describe your health condition. Write them down, ask what they mean, then put the information in your own words.

Medication can be used appropriately for a number of reasons. These include:

1. Curing a condition, as in the use of antibiotics for the treatment of an infection;

2. Treating symptoms, as in pain therapy;

3. Controlling a disease without curing it, as with high blood pressure or asthma therapy;

4. Slowing or arresting the course of a disease, as in the treatment of some types of arthritis or cancer.

Once you understand your condition well enough to describe it accurately to another person, you have a good grasp of what is really going on. Knowing what health problem you have will give you a better idea of why it is being treated in the way it is. It should also clear up doubts about why certain things have not been done. The best way for you to clear the air is also the easiest: ask the prescriber for more information.

Don't feel self-conscious writing down what is said. Most people forget at least half of what a prescriber says even before leaving the office. It is your right and responsibility to ask for and get information about your personal health.

What is the Expected Outcome?

Next, learn the *expected outcome* of your therapy. You know a description of the health condition you have. Now you need to find out what to expect from the recommended therapy. It is important to know both the condi-

tion being treated and the expected outcome of the treatment. How long the medication must be taken depends
on both of these factors. Success of the therapy also
affects the duration of treatment. If the treatment is
not achieving the desired goal, it is changed. It may be
lengthened. The dose may be increased. A different medication may need to be added or substituted. Find out the
answers to questions like:

Will you be cured?

Will the symptoms be controlled?

Will your health gradually fail?

How long will you be taking the medication?

Obviously there are no guarantees as far as outcome is
concerned, but get the doctor's best estimate on what to
expect and when to expect it.

The Name of the Medication

Now is when you should learn the *medication name.* Have
it written down and pronounced for you. Don't be coy,
you can learn "that awful long drug name." Some day
you may need to tell someone about the medication you
take. Find out if you are learning the brand or generic
name. Every medication product has a generic name and
some also have brand names. This can be confusing for
health professionals so you, too, may sometimes be
bewildered. Here is an explanation that may help to
demystify medication names.

Medications have a *chemical* name or description. This is usually meaningful for medicinal chemists, but not something most people would remember or use on a daily basis. Beside their chemical description, medications are assigned a *generic* name. All products that contain a particular chemical will be called by the established generic name. Some manufacturers make the medication and give it a special or *brand* name. This is particularly true if the manufacturer is the one that developed the chemical. Here's an example:

The product described chemically as 3,3 Dimethyl-7-oxo-6-[(phenoxyacetyl)amino]-4-thia-1-azabicyclo[3.2.0] heptane-2-carboxylic acid; or 6-phenoxyacetamido-penicillanic acid is the product we know as Penicillin V. Penicillin V is the generic name. The potassium salt of this medication is more familiar as Ledercillin. Ledercillin is the registered trademark of Lederle Laboratories.

Once you know why you are taking the medication, the expected outcome or what the medication is supposed to do, and its name, you have a great foundation on which to build. However, there's more to learn. You can continue to increase your medication information.

How Much?

What is the *dose* of medication you have been told to take? How much of the medication are you taking? The dose can be indicated in measures of weight such as mg   =   milligrams

mcg   =   micrograms

g   =   grams

Dose is sometimes expressed in measures of volume like

ml = milliliter

teaspoonsful = 5 ml

tablespoonsful = 15 ml

drops, droppersful, scoopsful

You may also see doses described as percentages and mEq = milliEquivalents. These are essentially measures of strength.

The only time you would not see one of these abbreviations is when the medication is a combination of several drugs. Multiple drugs in a single dosage form are frequently seen with cold preparations, and occasionally with other products such as blood pressure medicines. For example, Actifed, registered trademark of the Burroughs Wellcome Company, has two medications in each tablet in addition to inert or inactive ingredients. Combination products do not usually have a strength notation.

Learn how many units are in your standard dose. For example, you should be able to say, "Each tablet has 250 mg and I take two tablets to make each dose. This means I take 500 mg for each dose."

For How Long?

Find out the expected *duration of therapy*. Although it is similar to "expected outcome," duration of therapy refers to how long the medication is to be taken. This may be short-term as with antibiotics or "for the rest of your life" as with medications used to treat conditions like thyroid disorders.

How Often?

It is important to know how often the medication is to be taken or used. Find out specifically what the directions mean. Does three times a day mean once every 8 hours or one dose with each of three meals? A study of doctors, nurses, and pharmacists showed little agreement on the meaning of prescription directions. Be sure to ask what *your* prescriber and pharmacist believe you should do. Ask that this information be put on the prescription and prescription label. For example, the directions "Take one tablet four times a day 1 hour before meals and at bedtime" are much clearer than directions that say simply "Take one tablet four times a day."

Working New Medications Into Your Existing Routine

Be sure to let the prescriber know what your medication regimen is presently like. If you already have four medication dosing times each day, find out if the new medicine can be worked into your existing schedule. Try to keep your medication regimen or schedule as simple as possible. Again, this means you'll have to be your own advocate or take a friend with you to appointments to help. Prescribers can only help if you let them know your concerns.

When You Realize You've Missed a Dose

Ask your pharmacist what to do if you miss a dose of a particular medication. The answer may be different for each of the medications you take. Write down the answer.

What Could Go Wrong?

You already know the possible beneficial effects of your medication. What *side effects* should you be watching for? Many of you have read drug information books in which hundreds of side effects were listed for every product. These lists reflect every complaint the participants in the drug studies experienced. For example, if Mr. Finn is in a drug study for a blood pressure medicine and gets constipated, then constipation may appear on the complete side effects list even if Mr. Finn was the only one to become constipated.

What should be more useful to you than these long lists is to know first what the most likely side effects are for each of your medications. Then, you can ask what less frequent events could occur. For example, aspirin can cause nausea and stomach upset. Less frequently, it can cause significant gastrointestinal bleeding. The signs of such bleeding are vomiting coffee ground-like material or red blood or passing black tarry stools. That's worth knowing.

Obviously, learning side effects could become quite a task. Ask your pharmacist for patient information leaflets or for a copy of information about your medication from the book *United States Pharmacist Dispensing Information* (USP DI) *Advice for the Patient*. These sources condense the information so it contains the most important facts about your medications. Unless you have a health care or scientific background, I doubt the *Physicians' Desk Reference* (PDR) or books like it are good information sources for you.

Two excellent sources of medication information are: *About Your Medicine* (from USP) and *The Pill Book* (from Bantam). Many pharmacies keep these books on hand for their patrons.

Interactions

Is there a problem with *one of your medications interacting with another medication you are taking?* This is an area in which you must almost entirely depend on your pharmacist and prescriber. Unless these members of your health care team know *all* the medications you are taking, they cannot help to protect you from these problems. You'll want to find out right away if new medication can be taken with your existing regimen. Again, express to the prescriber any concerns you have about your regimen getting too complicated to manage. It has been shown that the more medications you take, the higher your risk of interactions between your medications.

Remember that alcohol and nicotine are both drugs and can interact with medications. Ask your prescriber how much alcohol you can drink while you are taking medication. Be sure the physician knows you use tobacco products if that is the case.

If you experience new problems soon after beginning therapy with a new medication, contact your pharmacist or prescriber. They can help you determine whether it is a side effect, interaction, or unrelated condition.

Monitoring

Are there any *special instructions* related to your medication? Does it have to be *monitored* in any special way? Find out what the tests and monitors are for your medications. Do you need routine blood pressure or blood glucose checks? Eye exams? Hearing evaluations? Find out how frequently they should be performed. The easiest way to remember these instructions will be to write them down.

Storing Your Medicines

What *storage conditions* are suggested for your medications? See Chapter 19 for a full definition of what accepted storage temperatures are. In general, cool, dry places are best for medicine, but this can vary.

Learning: A Lifetime Habit

Give yourself plenty of time to learn these things. Obviously, the more medications you are taking the more you will be learning at each step. Repetition will help a great deal, so talk about the medication facts you have learned. Because it would be nice to have a worksheet to use in keeping track of your progress, one is included. You can use it as a guide for the information you put in your medication diary. Chapter 7 details the medication diary. Be sure to also make a worksheet for each of your non-prescription medications. The main thing is to get started and keep working at it.

Another Way to Preserve the Facts

In addition to the worksheet, an excellent way to keep your medication information together is to buy a small bound ledger book at your pharmacy or office supply store and record everything there. You can use it to keep track of appointments, the starting date of medicines, outcome, questions for your health care team, laboratory data and so on. It is compact and can help you keep from losing the information you will need to participate in your health care. The value of a medication ledger or diary is discussed further in Chapter 7.

Medication Learning Plan Worksheet

Your name:

Date begun:

Indication or reason for taking this medication:

Expected outcome of therapy:

Medication name (generic and brand):

Dose taken:

Schedule of doses:

Expected duration of therapy:

Possible side effects:

Interactions to watch for:

Special instructions:

Things to monitor:

Storage:

If the dose or schedule of doses changes, draw a single line through the outdated information. Then write the new information *and* the date it became effective.

Chapter 6

Nonprescription Medications

This chapter focuses on medications that are available without a prescription. You will see how these "over the counter" (OTC) products get their status from the FDA and some concerns associated with making medications available without a prescription. You will learn to evaluate your health conditions and needs. This self-evaluation will help you determine when it is safe to self-medicate and when you should see your doctor or pharmacist. The roles of doctors and pharmacists in self-medicating are explained. You will be given guidelines useful for choosing OTC products. Included also is a brief discussion of vitamins and of natural and organic products.

Qualifying as an OTC Medication

Medications that qualify for nonprescription status have special characteristics.

1. They are relatively safe. Experts at the Food and Drug Administration (FDA) see them as having low potential for abuse and as unlikely to be habit forming.

2. They can be administered safely without professional supervision.

3. The condition being treated can be self-diagnosed.

4. It is possible to create labeling that allows patients to safely use the medication.

5. Side effects are minor.

The U.S. government and its agencies like the FDA are moving to make more medications available without prescriptions. This will have the advantage of allowing people even greater opportunities to self-prescribe and self-medicate. It will also increase each consumer's responsibility to find out whether products are appropriate for him or her to use. Your unique set of health conditions and prescription medications mean you must determine if an OTC medication is safe for *you*.

Shortcomings of Self-Medicating

The plan to make more products available without a prescription is based on some assumptions which may or may not be entirely correct or safe.

1. It is assumed that people are quite sophisticated in their knowledge of disease states and appropriate therapies for them. This includes the ability to determine the correct medication, dose, and duration of therapy.

2. It is assumed that people will reassess their medical conditions regularly and be able to determine accurately whether the therapy is working.

3. It is assumed that people will seek medical help when it should be sought.

4. Most importantly, it is assumed that the nonprescription (OTC) medication doesn't interact with the patient's prescribed medications or make his or her medical conditions worse.

When is it Appropriate to Use an OTC Medication?

Your medication regimen consists of all the medicines you take or use including oral, topical, eye, ear, rectal, and injectable medications. People over age 65 generally find that their medication regimens grow as time goes by. A major contributor to this complexity comes from the use of OTC products. The elderly make up approximately 12 percent of the U.S. population (Developments in Aging, 1988), but they purchase about 25 percent of all OTC products (American Medical Association White Paper, 1990).

There are several avenues of approach to self-medication with OTC medications. By performing a self-assessment, you may determine that an OTC medication is appropriate for your condition. Another way is to contact your pharmacist for advice on self-medicating. A third alternative is to contact your physician. Let's examine each in turn.

Self-Assessment of Your Health Problems

To determine whether it is safe to self-medicate a health problem, interview yourself. Ask yourself questions from this list about your particular situation.

1. What exactly is your complaint? What are your symptoms? Do you know what's causing them?

2. Have you ever experienced the condition or anything like it before? If so, what did you do then? What was the outcome?

3. When did you first notice the problem? Can you relate the onset of the symptoms to any other event?

4. Does it sometimes get better or worse at different times of the day, like at nighttime or after meals?

5. What have you done about the problem so far? What helped? What made it worse?

6. Who have you consulted for advice?

Let me give you an example of how using this self-assessment can help you improve your ability to correctly identify and solve health problems.

A Sudden Change of Health

Mrs. Diske follows the interview format for self-assessment. She wants to determine if it will be safe and effective to self-medicate.

1. Mrs. Diske's complaint is severe shortness of breath. She is at a loss to explain the source of her problem. She has no other symptoms such as a runny nose or chest pain.

2. She has never experienced similar symptoms.

3. She noticed a gradual onset of shortness of breath in just the past 2 weeks. Actually, this all seemed to begin following her last medication change. At that time, she began medication therapy for high blood pressure.

4. There doesn't seem to be a pattern of when the symptoms are worse.

5. So far she has tried humidifying the air in her bedroom with no improvement in her symptoms. She is now quite concerned that she might have a serious condition.

6. She discussed the matter with friends and family. One of them suggested she buy an OTC oral inhaler marketed for asthma.

Mrs. Diske developed new, serious symptoms within several weeks of changing her prescription medications. Her self-assessment told her to check with her doctor. Her doctor saw her right away and discontinued the new blood pressure medicine. Her symptoms went away. She was monitored for further problems. Mrs. Diske realized that using an OTC medication in this situation might mask or prolong the condition and put her health in danger.

It's not always easy for you to determine whether you should use an OTC medication or see your doctor. Here are some guidelines for deciding. Used in combination with the self-assessment, they provide you with the information you need to make an informed decision about self-medicating.

When to See the Doctor

You should see your doctor when any of the following situations occur.

1. When you experience a new and serious health problem with sudden onset or with severe symptoms.

2. If you are in poor overall health.

3. If your problem began within several weeks of starting a new medication or other therapy or of getting a new diagnosis.

4. When the problem is one that you have been told to watch for by a member of your health care team.

The Doctor Advises an OTC Medication

Discussion with your doctor may result in the recommendation of an OTC product. For example, if you have been worried by some chest pain, it is reasonable to see your doctor. There are several potential causes of this pain and your doctor can diagnose it. In some cases, the diagnosis will be hiatal hernia or indigestion. Your doctor might recommend an OTC antacid with specific suggestions as to how much and how frequently you should take it.

It is important to realize that OTC products suggested for you by your doctor are part of your medication regimen. You need to get instructions for their use as if they were prescription drugs. Your doctor should be notified if you alter the directions or decide to discontinue the medication.

What the Pharmacist Can Do to Help

Sometimes you may be reasonably sure that you do not need to see a doctor. Nonetheless, you may feel the need for advice other than that you get from friends or family. Consider your family pharmacist.

Your pharmacist can assist you in deciding whether it is safe for you to self-medicate and help you choose an appropriate OTC product. The pharmacist does these things by:

1. Helping you determine the exact nature of your ailment.

2. Steering you to a doctor when that seems prudent.

3. Helping you choose a product that will adequately treat your ailment without exposing you to unneeded medications.

4. Helping you select the best product for the situation at the best price.

5. Helping you decide when another medication is *not* needed.

6. Helping you determine whether a product you already have at home will help treat the current situation.

Picture Mrs. Garden repotting her houseplants without wearing gloves. When she finishes, her hands are a mess. There is no way she can go to the Senior Center with her hands looking like that. When repeated scrubbing with soap and water doesn't work, she digs around under the sink and finds a solvent for cleaning spots on the garage floor. In desperation, she tries the solvent. It gets most of the dirt off, but her hands begin to redden and feel raw.

Mrs. Garden is not quite sure how serious her problem is. She drops by the pharmacy to get some advice. Her pharmacist listens to the story, checks her profile for current medical conditions, medications, and allergies. Mrs. Garden has diabetes for which she takes oral medication and checks her blood glucose at home once a week. She also takes a diuretic (water pill) for blood pressure control. She is allergic to sulfa drugs.

Her skin is not painful or blistered. Her hands have not swollen nor has the redness become more intense. The incident occurred in the middle of the week, so if the condition worsens she will still be able to catch her doctor in the office before the weekend.

Since Mrs. Garden otherwise feels well, her pharmacist suggests that she apply Eucerin cream (Registered trademark of Beiersdorf, Inc.) several times daily to moisturize her hands. Her pharmacist explains that the redness may persist for a week and that the cream has no medications added to it and will not interfere with her prescription medications. Her pharmacist suggests she check her blood glucose daily for the next week to determine if it is being affected by the injury. If abnormal readings are obtained, she should contact her doctor. She is also instructed that if the redness becomes more intense or if she experiences pain, swelling, blistering, or numbness, she should contact her doctor at once.

Though Mrs. Garden's initial decision to apply the solvent to her hands was a poor one, she used her resources well in resolving the problem. She was able to get help from her pharmacist in sorting out the important factors and the possible treatment of the condition. There were many products available to treat skin conditions, but Mrs. Garden needed a product that would treat her condition without interfering with her prescription medication.

Choosing an OTC Medication

Once you alone or in combination with your doctor or pharmacist have decided to use an OTC product, the task of choosing the right one begins. You probably have been exposed to a great deal of marketing of OTC products. This is bound to play some role in your purchase and use of an OTC product. Product advertising relies heavily on playing up one attractive aspect of the product while ignoring possible risks. As the informed consumer, you must remember that risks and benefits occur together whenever medications are taken. Manufacturers and packagers of OTC products can mislead you by pretty packaging, aligning the product with admired female or male traits or noted personalities, or by implying that use of the product will bring youth and vitality. Awareness of this persuasion can be helpful in keeping you from purchasing and using a product that is not appropriate for your situation.

Buy Only What You Need

A great number of OTC products are available. As a matter of fact, there may be too many products with too many medications in them. This sounds strange until it is explained. If you get a cold with runny nose and cough, the symptoms you want to treat are runny nose and cough. Many products, for example, those advertised to treat colds, have multiple active ingredients. They treat cough, cold, fever, allergy and so on. The temptation is to buy a product that does everything. Good sense should dictate that you don't treat symptoms you don't have.

Buy the Product Not the Package

Packaging is designed to induce you to buy a product. Try to view the product in terms of what it is intended to do and not just how the product is presented. Do not buy a product because it is attractively packaged. Do not buy more of a product than you really need. As you know, packages of a larger quantity are generally less expensive per unit. Of course, if you won't use all of a product, then you haven't saved money. Consider also whether having larger amounts of medication around the house might present a hazard. The section in Chapter 12 on poison prevention packaging addresses this issue in depth.

Compare Prices

The products you want will probably be available from several manufacturers. Costs will be affected by such things as being the "innovator" product (first one made), fancy packaging, and the degree to which the product is marketed in the media. If you are faithful to a particular brand and it has worked for you in the past, then your decision is made. You buy "your" brand. Once you've decided a particular medication is safe and appropriate for you, compare the prices that several manufacturers are charging for that product. As seasoned shoppers know, price comparison can be difficult, so don't be shy about asking for help from store employees in determining costs per dose.

Read Labels

The goal of this book is not to have you memorize a great number of facts, it is to help you recognize and utilize your resources and to successfully solve the problems related to health and medications with which you are confronted. In the case of purchasing a new OTC medication, the best way to get a safe and effective product will be to read the label before you buy. By careful reading, you may find, for example, that two OTC products used for the same ailment have nearly the same ingredients. You may be able to save money by buying the less expensive product. The label may also tell you if you have a condition that would be worsened by the product.

Ask Your Pharmacist

OTC labels, while quite extensive, may not contain all the information you need for a wise decision. Your pharmacist can help.

Your prescription medications may interact with the OTC medication. Even the most harmless OTC product can create problems if combined with the wrong prescription medication. Numerous interactions are possible with nearly every category of medicine. For example, ibuprofen works against some blood pressure medicines. Antacids cannot be taken within an hour of certain antibiotics. It is also easy to mix two OTC medications in a way that is harmful or illogical. The best way to be certain is to ask your pharmacist about interactions. For this reason, it is a good idea to purchase your OTC products at the same pharmacy that fills your prescriptions.

Two sets of products in the OTC section have disputed benefits. One is vitamins and minerals the other "natural" and organic products.

Vitamins and Minerals

Popular with the public, vitamins and mineral supplements are taken for proven and unproven reasons. A variety of vitamins in many strengths and combinations can be found in pharmacies, supermarkets, and natural food stores, to mention only a few sources. Your pharmacist and local dietician have lists of the U.S. Recommended Daily Allowance (RDA) for vitamins. Experts at the National Academy of Sciences determine the RDA, not special interest groups or manufacturers. When you read or hear information about vitamins, be sure to consider the source. A considerable number of untrained, unqualified people and publications are busily offering advice about vitamins that has questionable value.

Minerals such as calcium, iron, iodine, zinc, copper, magnesium, and phosphorus also have U.S. RDAs established for them. Others like selenium, fluoride, chromium, and molybdenum have not currently had RDAs determined. Since there is no RDA, it is difficult to decide what dose is right for you. The dose of a product containing vitamins or minerals may be far greater or less than the RDA. Read labels carefully to determine this.

Minerals may be available in several forms or salts. Look for the amount of available mineral content when purchasing mineral supplements. For example, calcium is available as carbonate, phosphate, and gluconate salts. Fewer tablets of the carbonate preparation must be taken to get the recommended 1000 mg of calcium per day. A similar situation exists with iron supplements. Again, read the label and ask for assistance to keep from buying the wrong product.

Your Maximum Should Be the Recommended Daily Allowance

Pharmacists are taught to encourage people to achieve adequate vitamin and mineral intake through their diet. Nonetheless, it is often reasonable for a person who does not eat well to consider taking a multiple vitamin and mineral supplement. Most pharmacists believe that anytime a person thinks he or she needs more than the RDA of vitamins, that person should be seen by a doctor for assessment. The health concern that causes a person to seek to "megadose" vitamins may reflect the presence of a serious medical condition.

OTC vitamins are sold as nutritional supplements and not as medications to treat an abnormal condition. Before using vitamins as medication therapy for some condition or in amounts that exceed the RDA, consult a doctor. Emergency rooms occasionally must treat people for the effects of excessive vitamin intake. Vitamins can and do interact with medications. They can cause toxicity and "withdrawal" type syndromes on discontinuation of high doses.

The message is: *more is not necessarily better.* OTC vitamins are to be consumed in moderation both for your health and pocketbook.

Natural and Organic Products

A word or two about "natural" products. The term "natural" is loosely defined if at all. Natural can mean from naturally occurring sources, but in that case it would cover nearly everything. Natural may also mean produced without certain chemical interventions. It's hard to say what the packager of such a product is actually claiming. Based on FDA criteria, a product sold in the United States and labeled to contain 50 mg of a medication will contain 50 mg of that substance, regardless of the source or process of manufacture. It may be that "natural" is a synonym for "needlessly expensive." No scientific information shows "natural" products to be superior to other types of products.

Also, there are currently no legal requirements that help to define "organically grown" products. Because there is no standardization of this category of products, it is also impossible to tell how they may be superior or inferior to similar products. They too are often high priced.

Summary

OTC medications can be useful and inexpensive products for treating minor ailments. In the United States, OTC medications include only what the government believes can be safely used by conscientious consumers. The therapeutic effectiveness of these products is not an issue; they are medications and have all the potential to help or harm that other medications do.

The trend toward more OTC medications puts you in a position of tremendous responsibility. Deciding when and how to use these valuable products is an important skill for you to learn. This underscores the importance of you becoming a competent, informed member of your health care team. You need to know which members of the team are best qualified to assist in any particular health situation. Regarding OTC medication use, this means primarily your pharmacist and doctor.

Chapter 7

Keeping A Medication Diary

One of the best ways to monitor your progress on medication is with a simple medication diary. Keeping track of side effects; symptoms; monitors such as blood pressure, pulse, blood glucose; and medication names and doses can be valuable. It helps you retrieve important information related to your medications. Also, by writing down medication-related information or events along with the dates that they occur, you can create an accurate picture of how well you fare on your medication therapy.

How to Start Your Medication Diary

General Information

1. Buy a hardbound ledger book from a stationary or office supply store or pharmacy. This ledger will help you keep all the information in one place and assure you that no pages get misplaced.

2. Specify all who are involved in your care and their telephone numbers.

3. Record all significant changes in your health and living status.

4. Record the expected outcomes from therapy.

5. Date every entry you make in the diary.

6. Write in ink, and indicate an error by drawing a single line through the entry. Never erase anything you write in the diary; it may be useful to you later.

Setting Up Your Diary

You can set the diary up in the following way:

Page 1   Your full name

Your signature

The date

Your street and mailing addresses

Your phone number (including area code)

Your birthdate

Any medication allergy, when it occurred and what reaction you experienced

Last tetanus vaccination, if any

Year of pneumonia vaccine, if any

State whether you get yearly flu shots

Page 2   Enter the names and telephone numbers of your health care team members. You can tape their business cards on this page if you find this more convenient.

Page 3   List all the medical conditions for which you have ever been treated. Circle the conditions for which you are now being actively treated.

Page 4   List any special equipment you require and useful details about it such as size, brand, and your supplier's name and telephone number. For example:

nebulizer

ostomy products

incontinence products

pessary

urinary catheter and bags

central venous catheter

peripheral venous access

Page 5   Begin your medication information. Save two pages for each medication. You've got lots of pages to work with. Always start a diary entry by writing the day's date. Then write down:

the medication name,

why you are taking the medication,

the strength of each tablet or capsule,

how often and how many you take each day.

When a change occurs, draw a single line through the original information and tell what happened. For example, if the dose was changed, write "dose changed" and the date the change occurred. If a medication was discontinued, write "prescriber stopped this" and the date. Try to be brief but clear in your explanations. Any time your prescriber changes the therapy, update that page and *date* it. If for some reason *you* change the therapy, write down the change you made and the date you made it. You should explain this in the "diary" part of your book.

Continue entering medication information until you have two pages devoted to each of your current medications including products for eyes, ears, skin, and nonprescription medications.

Skip 10 or 15 pages, leaving them blank. You can use these for new medications that may be prescribed in the future. You will also need pages to use as worksheets for going to the doctor and for hospital or nursing home discharge information. More information about these worksheets appears in Chapters 14 and 16.

The Diary Part of Your Medication Diary

Now you are ready to begin the diary portion of your book. Write the date on a page and make an entry about how you are feeling on your current therapy. This is called the baseline. No one but you will probably ever read this book so don't feel shy about what you reveal. An example of an entry is:

> January 14, 1993. Feel pretty good today. Some joint pain, but better since medication was changed last week. I finally got over the diarrhea.

In the diary portion, be sure to record information and questions you might want to discuss with your doctor when you next have an appointment. Try to make at least two entries in the medication diary a week.

This diary can be the record of your health. It will give you an idea of how things are really progressing. For example, was it 10 days ago or 3 weeks ago that you fell? Did you have an upset stomach before you started taking that new medication or did it begin afterward? Your diary can also provide a valuable tool for your prescriber, nurse, or pharmacist as they help you maintain your good health.

Chapter 8

Skills Needed For
Medication Management

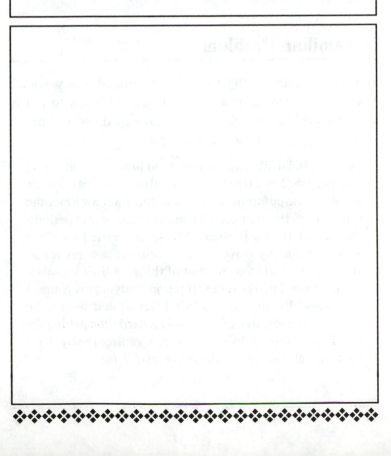

The outlook for people with health problems has never been brighter. New medications are being discovered and developed every day. Each person's responsibility in learning to manage these medications is great. Fortunately, there are abundant sources of help in this endeavor. This chapter will identify and review some basic problem solving strategies, skills, and abilities needed for safe and effective medication management. It will remind you of the experts who can provide you with sound information. Finally, it will describe skills and behaviors you can develop that will help you succeed as a medication manager.

A Familiar Problem

In today's world we all contend with some things we don't necessarily know a great deal about. We learn to apply existing problem-solving techniques to these unknown areas. Here is a personal example:

> I own a car. I drive it and understand how it should sound and behave. The extent of my attention to the car usually involves just pumping fuel into it. But I am aware of the other things the car needs. I own a tire gauge and periodically check the air pressure. I have the desired numbers written inside my glove compartment for easy reference. It makes me feel in command of things, a little bit sassy, in fact, when I'm out at the air pump studying my gauge. I also know that the car has "vital fluids" that need to be checked periodically. Since I have a hard time getting the hood open and I don't want to risk getting greasy, I get someone else to check these things for me.

My point here is that while I don't do my car's maintenance all myself, I do take responsibility for getting it done.

I also take action when my car does something undesirable or unexpected. If it continues to do it or if the symptoms are severe enough, like the engine conks out entirely, I seek professional help. I've been pretty lucky in finding mechanics who understand me and what I want for my car. I present the problem. My mechanic diagnoses it in terms of automotive workings. We decide together how to handle the repairs. I am either satisfied with the work, or I go back to the mechanic and we try again.

Cars and their workings and failures are familiar to most of us. We have been struggling and tinkering with them since we were teenagers. However, we usually learn about health problems and how to manage them later in our lives. Our juvenile ailments were handled by parents and doctors. Amazingly, we may feel more at home talking to the car mechanic than our doctor, nurse, or pharmacist. While the facts about car maintenance may not help you manage your medication, the same problem-solving skills apply.

Problem Solving

There's a logical sequence of thoughts you can apply when you encounter problems of any kind, including those involved with medication management. This is the sequence:

1. List all the details you know about the problem. Piece together the facts you have and try to identify the actual problem.

2. Determine if your problem is similar to any problem you have previously experienced. If so, review how the situations are similar and how they differ. Recall how you resolved the previous problem.

3. Determine a course of action to alter the problem. If an expert should be consulted, decide which one.

4. Undertake your course of action and keep good records of your endeavor. This way you will be able to learn something from the problem regardless of whether you choose a successful path.

5. Evaluate the results. If your plan did not succeed, start over at the first step.

Regardless of the type of problem you encounter, you will need some knowledge, skills, and abilities particular to that problem in order to implement your solution.

Skills and Abilities for Medication Taking

Many people have studied medication-taking behavior. It can be broken down into a few elements that describe the skills and abilities you need to be safe and effective in this important task. These are:

1. The ability to understand and remember the nature of the medication regimen.

2. The motivation to comply with the therapy recommendations by following through in taking the medications and keeping appointments with the health care team.

3. The knowledge that supports your reason and method for using the medication.

4. The skills to perform the tasks needed for taking the medication properly. These include the skills to organize the regimen so the right medication gets taken on schedule. It also means opening and closing the containers, removing tablets, and taking them. These skills also include proper storage, refilling, and discontinuing medications as ordered.

By evaluating each of these four elements, you can determine the degree of self-administration of medication that you can handle safely and effectively.

Memory

The failure of a individual's short-term memory can be a problem when it comes to managing medication. Imagine not being able to remember what happened 5 minutes ago. This can lead to doubled or missed doses of medication. Long-term memory failure can cause an individual to forget what the therapy is for, therefore eliminating the motivation to take the medication. Either problem could make a person a poor manager and reporter of their health-related problems. In Chapter 18, there are some suggestions for overcoming these handicaps.

Motivation

The motivation to comply with your medication regimen can be adversely affected by such problems as:

1. Depression

2. Uncertainty and misunderstanding

3. Financial worries

4. Lack of confidence

5. Side effects

6. Social or cultural taboos

Some examples of statements made by patients with faltering motivation are:

"Oh, what's the use. I'm dying anyway."

"I'm not sure I should be taking hormones. I heard somewhere . . ."

"I feel fine. Anyway, these are too expensive for me to buy every month."

"I feel lousy so I don't get up for every dose."

"I think this pill is messing up my sexual relations, so which is worse? The condition I'm treating or the one caused by the treatment?"

"People in my culture don't take your cures."

Researchers have found that poor motivation is hard to modify. They do make some suggestions for those who would help motivate themselves or another person. They suggest:

1. Remove all the obstacles to compliance that can be identified.

2. Support your own or the other person's compliance.

3. Seek out or provide ongoing teaching and contact.

Besides cheering ourselves or another person on for compliance, we have to minimize the obstacles to it. This means trying to make sure that functional things such as reading prescription labels, opening the containers, remembering each dose, and being able to get to the pharmacy and prescriber for refills and check ups are possible. It means going to members of the health care team with concerns and questions. For yourself, it may mean facing up to the personal reasons for low motivation.

Knowledge

Knowledge about health and disease supports your choice to take your medication. Your ability to learn new information and skills is what helps keep you independent. You've been learning, interpreting, and remembering information all your life. To have lived so long, you must be fairly good at it. Perhaps you just haven't thought much lately about learning. If you are faced with managing medications, however, you'll find yourself learning all the time. Maintaining a medication diary, described in Chapter 7, is one easy way to get back into some structured learning habits.

If you've gotten out of the habit of consciously learning new things, but need to do so now, start slowly, pace yourself, and give yourself pats on the back. You deserve it for getting started again!

The content in Chapter 5 helps you develop a system for learning more about your medication.

Functional Skills and Abilities

Even if you know all about your medications, you will still need a few additional skills and abilities. These include vision for reading; hearing for directions and telephoning; and dexterity for packaging, unpackaging, and storing medication.

A Simple Quiz

It is important to identify *your* skills for medication taking. Such identification is fairly simple. The following five-part quiz will reveal many of your strengths. Once you have completed the quiz, you can read what your answers might mean.

1. Open and close a prescription vial with a safety cap on it. Time yourself. Don't give up. How long did it take to complete the task?

2. Open and close a prescription vial with a nonsafety cap on it. Again, time yourself. How long did it take?

3. Remove two tablets from a prescription vial containing 30 or more tablets. What difficulties did you experience? Did any tablets spill out?

4. Read aloud the entire directions from the labels of two of your prescription vials. Explain to someone else what the directions mean.

5. Describe your entire medicine schedule.

You will need to be able to open either the safety or nonsafety caps and complete the other three tasks to be totally and completely independent in administering your own medicine.

Interpreting Your Results

The question of opening and closing vials indicates whether you have the strength and manual dexterity to open and close the vials and remove the tablets. Removing the tablets will show if you have a tremor or some other problem and, if so, how severe.

Reading instructions aloud will reveal whether you need glasses to read the label and whether you understand that the vial must be turned to read the entire directions. You'll also demonstrate that you can read English in the print size on the prescription label.

Your ability to paraphrase the directions will show you understand what you have to do to correctly schedule and take the medicine. Finally, the quiz shows how well you use your resources and your creativity. Unfortunately, it cannot tell if you actually want to or will comply with the therapy.

If you have some functional shortcomings, don't despair, a solution may be available from a member of your health care team. Assessing your skills and abilities to manage medication should tell you whether you are safe to independently manage your medicine or whether you should seek assistance in this task.

By taking the quiz, you have taken an important step toward identifying where help is needed. More important than being perfect is recognizing your strengths and resources and using them to overcome any weaknesses.

Chapter 9

Taking the Medication

We still have to deal with the practical matter of taking the medication. Even if you are convinced of the benefits and are ready, willing, and able to confront medication therapy, the nagging problem remains of actually taking the medication. This chapter will describe how a medication schedule can be tailored to your lifestyle. Finally, the actual steps to follow when taking medication of all kinds will be introduced.

Medication management is best accomplished with a well thought out system. The system should be simple. It needs to be something that makes sense to *you* and which you could explain to members of your health care team. It should be easy enough that you can do it even on your worst days. Ideally, it should fit right into your daily routine.

Developing Your System

Here is one approach to adapting your medication schedule to fit your personal habits.

1. Make a calendar of your routine activities. Write down what you normally do each day. What time you rise, eat, nap, and so on. To this, add a list of things you sometimes do, for example, Thursday afternoon bridge game.

2. Make a list of your medications and when they should be taken. Note any restrictions on when they can be taken such as on an empty stomach or with food.

3. Next, set up a written schedule for your daily medications. Get your pharmacist to help you, if necessary. Find out how much leeway you have on the time each dose must be taken. It is helpful to know whether the medication can be given an hour early or late without problems. This way you'll know how rigid your medication schedule is.

4. Remember, you must manage all your dosage forms. Not all of what you may be asked to take will come in tablet or capsule form. You must also create a system that allows you to efficiently manage medication when it comes as:

a. oral liquids;

b. powders for dissolution;

c. topical preparations such as creams, lotions, ointments, patches, and films;

d. rectal or vaginal creams or suppositories;

e. injectable substances and the associated equipment for them like swabs and syringes;

f. monitoring materials. The strips and other equipment for monitoring blood or urine glucose and urine ketones are as important to the success of therapy as the medications themselves.

g. eye (ophthalmic) and ear (otic) products.

5. Try your schedule for a week or 10 days.

6. If you just can't live with your medication schedule, determine where you will have to make changes. If you need help "fine tuning" the schedule, call your doctor, nurse, or pharmacist. Your goal is to create a medication administration schedule that doesn't control your life but does get the desired benefits of the treatment. Several types of medication schedules are shown below.

Schedule 1

MEDICATION NAME AND STRENGTH	TIME OF DAY TO TAKE DOSE			
	Morning	Noon	Supper	Bedtime
Aaaaa 200 mg	1 tablet	—	—	—
Bbbbb 0.25 mg	1 capsule	—	—	—
Ccccc 40 mg	1 tablet	—	1 tablet	—
Ddddd 25 mg	—	—	—	2 tablets

Schedule 2

TIME OF DAY	MEDICATION TAKEN AT EACH TIME		
	Name	Strength	Number to Take
Morning	Aaaaa	200 mg	1 tablet
	Bbbbb	0.25 mg	1 capsule
	Ccccc	40 mg	1 tablet
Noon	— No Medications —		
Supper	Ccccc	40 mg	1 tablet
Bedtime	Ddddd	25 mg	2 tablets

Two types of medication schedules.

If you have relatively few medications and dosing times, you may be able to work out a medication schedule for yourself. Remember, however, that seeking the assistance of a member of your health care team is perfectly acceptable and is a good use of your resources. Devices that may help you manage your medications are described in Chapter 18.

Medication-Taking Techniques

General Procedures

To manage your own medications most effectively and safely, you will need:

1. Manual dexterity,

2. Good eyesight possibly supplemented by a magnifying lens,

3. A clean work area with bright lighting,

4. To wash your hands well for 15 seconds before administering any medication.

Oral Tablets and Capsules

With clean hands:

1. Select or measure the medication to be taken at the present dosing time.

2. Get a fresh glass of water to take with the medication.

3. Sit up, don't recline.

4. Take a swallow of water to lubricate your mouth, throat, and esophagus.

5. Put one pill in your mouth and then drink several swallows of water.

6. Repeat this process until you have taken all the tablets and/or capsules.

Powders and Liquids

Some of the powders commonly used include products to help control high cholesterol, psyllium products, and potassium supplements. Liquids requiring dilution before taking are often forms of potassium. The importance of taking these drugs correctly cannot be overemphasized. Some powders dissolved in an inadequate amount of liquid can cause intestinal blockage. Liquid medications containing potassium must be diluted correctly to minimize the risk of ulceration. To administer these products safely and effectively, follow these steps.

1. Measure 4 to 6 ounces of liquid into a large glass. Fill another glass with water to use as extra dilution following the medication.

2. Measure the powder or liquid to be taken in the dose. Stir it into the glass of liquid.

3. Drink a wetting gulp of water, then drink down the medication.

4. Follow this with your *full* glass of water.

Special Considerations for Orally Administered Medication

If your prescriber has you on fluid restriction, be sure to ask what changes to make in this procedure.

For people who have a problem swallowing thin liquids like water, tablets and capsules can be placed in food with the consistency of applesauce or pudding right before administration. Don't crush tablets or capsules without checking with your pharmacist to be sure it won't affect the potency or side effects of the medication. If further assistance seems necessary, have your doctor suggest a speech pathologist who can evaluate your swallow.

Ear Drops

Ears are located well for their primary purpose, hearing. Ears are somewhat inconveniently located when you wish to put medication in them. There are several ways to attack the problems of instilling ear drops.

The "Two Person Approach"

To instill ear drops into another person's ear do the following:

1. Roll the bottle of ear drops between your hands. This warms the drops and mixes the contents.

2. Have the patient lie on his or her side with the ear to be treated facing up.

3. Gently pull back on the ear lobe.

4. Fill the dropper with medication and hold the dropper over the ear canal. *Do not put the dropper in the ear itself.* Squeeze the prescribed number of drops into the ear.

5. Recap the bottle.

6. Have the person remain on his or her side for 2 to 5 minutes. Then repeat with the other ear if so directed.

Instilling Your Own Ear Drops

1. Stand or sit comfortably before a mirror in a well lighted room. Have a table or sink in front of you to steady yourself.

2. Roll the medication bottle between your hands to warm and mix the contents.

3. Open the bottle and fill the dropper. Tilt your head toward your shoulder so the ear to be treated is up. If it helps your balance, place your forearm flat on the sink or table and lean toward it.

4. Drop the prescribed number of drops into your ear. *Don't* put the dropper down into your ear.

5. Keep your ear facing the ceiling for 2 to 5 minutes. This gives the medication a chance to move all the way down to your eardrum.

6. Repeat with the other ear if directed.

Special Considerations When Using Ear Drops

In case you touch the dropper to your hand, head, tabletop or wherever, just wipe it clean with a tissue before putting it back in the bottle. This is to keep from contaminating the medication in the bottle.

Never heat ear drops by any method other that by rolling the bottle between your hands. It is easy to get the liquid too hot. This could damage your ear and cause the medication to break down.

Packing the ear with cotton once the drops are in is generally not necessary. Those few drops of medication are not going to gush out of the ear, but will move in the ear canal, coating it with medication as they go. That's good, but if your doctor tells you to use cotton, do so.

Oral Inhalers

Every package containing an oral inhaler has in it directions for use. These include diagrams and a step-by-step commentary on how to use the product correctly. You are supposed to receive this package insert *every* time you fill or refill a prescription for an oral inhaler. Studies have shown that people's technique in using oral inhalers tends to deteriorate over time. Because of this, you may want to review the package insert information each time you receive a refill. This returns us to the issue that repetition and reinforcement are helpful in maintaining good medication technique.

A Review of Oral Inhaler Technique

1. Shake the canister well.

2. Hold the mouthpiece in front of your open mouth with your teeth and tongue out of the way.

3. Lean your head back to open your airway.

4. Breathe out slowly, and while drawing in a slow, even, deep breath activate the canister by pressing down on it.

5. When the full breath has been drawn in, you should hold your breath for 10 seconds.

6. If a second puff is prescribed, it may be given after 1 minute by following the directions starting at step 1.

7. If your inhaled medication is a steroid such as beclomethasone, be sure to rinse your mouth with water after your doses. This will help keep you from getting an oral candida infection.

Common Problems in Administration

1. Failing to shake the canister for each puff can result in the delivery of an inaccurate dose. The medication is suspended in the aerosol liquid and settles between uses. To be assured of receiving the correct dose each time, the canister must be shaken to evenly disperse the medication within it.

2. Forgetting to hold your breath after inhaling the dose can keep medication from settling into the passageways of the lung where it will do the most good.

3. Not inhaling at the time the canister is depressed can result in most of a dose being deposited at the back of your mouth and wasted. Only medication that reaches your lungs will improve your breathing.

4. Holding the inhaler at the wrong distance from the mouth can keep the medication droplets from landing in the lungs where they are needed. The speed and size of the droplets are related to how far from your mouth the inhaler is held.

5. Not leaning your head back while inhaling the medicine makes medicine delivery less efficient. When you lean your head back as you inhale, the pathway is better for the medication droplets as they head for the lung.

6. Failing to periodically rinse the plastic holder to eliminate residue can keep you from getting the correct dosage. Doses may be wasted because they don't leave the inhaler at the right speed and particle size.

Improving Oral Inhaler Technique

The distance you hold the inhaler from your mouth really depends on you and how well you coordinate your breathing and activating the spray. Adjust your technique until you feel no powder (medication) on the back of your mouth and throat after you have inhaled. Any medication deposited there will not end up in your lungs where it is needed. There are devices available to make inhaling the medication more efficient. These devices are tube-shaped extenders or bags into which the dose can be sprayed before you inhale it. One of these devices is shown in the illustration on page 90. Ask your pharmacist to show you what he or she keeps in stock. The devices may require a doctor's prescription. They work well with correct instruction. Their disadvantages seem to be that they are bulky to carry around and that they require you to be able to learn new skills.

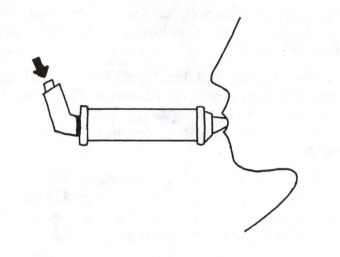

One extender device used with oral inhalers.

Ophthalmics: For the Eye

Eyedrops or ointments can present special problems for the elderly person. Any tremor can make it difficult to get the drop in the eye. Visual impairments can make it difficult to see what you're doing while instilling the drops. Here is a method that should be adaptable for most people.

Instilling Drops or Ointment into Your Own Eyes

1. Eye medications are sterile. Wash your hands each time before you administer the drops.

2. Work in a room with good lighting and a mirror that doesn't have to be held. Administration of eye medications is a two-handed procedure.

3. Using a finger of one hand, gently pull down on the lower eyelid to form a small pouch.

4. With the other hand squeeze one drop or about 1/8 inch of ointment into the pouch. Let go of the eyelid and just allow your eye to resume its normal activity. There is no need to rub the eye; your normal blinking will spread the medication.

5. Wait 10 seconds or so after putting in the first drop then put in another drop in the same eye if it is prescribed. Ointment is generally applied only once per dose.

The Two-Person Approach to Eye Drops or Ointment

It is probably most comfortable if you put in your own eye medications. For some people and at sometime for all people, this is not possible. In those cases, the person putting in the medication should follow the above directions and place the drop or strip of ointment in the lower pouch of the eye. It is best to try to put the drops in this way as there has been some concern that other methods might be harmful to the eye. Since it is difficult to judge the distance to another person's eye, putting the medication into the pouch may avoid injury or wasting medication.

Special Considerations with Eye Medications

Eyes cannot accommodate a lot of extra fluid, so if you put in two drops at once some medication may be flushed out of the eye and be wasted. Following the administration of eye drops, you can press gently for several seconds on the side of your nose where your glasses normally rest. This will keep the drops from being washed out of your eye and into your nose through a tiny canal. Incidentally, this is the route that tears take when you cry and make your nose run.

In many cases, a tremor can be conquered in this way. Stand in front of a wall-mounted mirror. Put your elbows on the wall at about shoulder height. You can then lean on your elbows or forearms to stabilize your hands. Put the eye drops or ointment in your eyes as directed. The bathroom mirror doesn't work well for this because the sink is in your way.

Skin Preparations

Skin preparations can be used as directed without a lot of fanfare. These preparations have relatively few cautions in their application.

1. Wash your hands and the site of application if appropriate.

2. Apply the medication sparingly to the clean skin unless otherwise directed.

3. Wash your hands afterwards.

4. Keep the medicine out of your eyes. Apply only to the areas directed. One of the daily applications should usually be right after your shower or bath when your skin is moist.

Vaginal Preparations

Vaginal medications can be inserted in the following ways:

1. The medication can be inserted while you are sitting on the toilet seat or standing if you are stable on your feet. You can stand and place one foot on the toilet or a stool as if you were climbing stairs. They can also be inserted while lying on a bed with your knees up.

2. Put the medication in the applicator. With vaginal suppositories, this involves unwrapping the suppository and loading it in the top of the applicator. For vaginal creams, the cap of the tube containing the cream is removed and the applicator is screwed on in its place. The applicator is filled to the appropriate level and the cream tube is removed.

3. Gently insert the applicator into your vagina. The medication should be placed as high in the vagina as is comfortable.

4. Wash the applicator under warm running water.

Ancillary Information

Generally, you will be instructed to insert vaginal medication at bedtime. This allows the medication time to dissolve and act in the vagina. When you are in an upright position, such as standing or sitting, the medication will tend to move downward and out of your body, thus taking it away from the area to be treated.

Rectal Preparations

To insert a medication rectally do the following:

1. Lie on your side with your bottom leg straight. Bend the other leg at the knee bringing it up toward your chest.

2. Remove the suppository from the wrapping.

3. If you wish, you may cover your finger tip with a latex finger cot, an object that looks like a single finger of a latex glove. Place the suppository on your fingertip and insert in your rectum. Generally, about an inch is far enough.

4. Relax a moment before getting up or you may have an urge to expel the suppository. Nonirritating lubricating jellies are available at your pharmacy. These may be used to coat the suppository or opening to the rectum to make inserting the suppository easier.

The technique is the same for rectal creams. They usually come in a tube with a slim attachment that you attach. Medication enters the rectum via the attachment when you squeeze the tube of medicine. Use great care with this setup so you don't damage the rectal tissue.

Injectables

Insulin

The subcutaneous injection of insulin along with special considerations for the diabetic are beyond the scope of this book. The care of diabetics has become a science unto itself and many excellent information sources can be obtained from health care team members with a special interest in this disease and by a referral from your doctor. A diabetic nurse educator at your local hospital is a good person with whom to begin your learning. Vast resources are available from the American Diabetes Association.

Papaverine

Papaverine is a medication which is used alone or in combination with phentolamine to help men achieve and sustain penile erection. The technique for administering this medication includes:

1. With clean hands, remove the metal protective cap on the vial to expose the rubber stopper. Swab the stopper with alcohol and allow to dry.

2. With a new needle and syringe, draw in the exact amount of air that will displace the fluid you draw out of the vial. Inject the air into the vial and withdraw the medication as shown in the illustration on page 96. Be careful not to touch the vial top or needle.

3. Wipe the injection site with alcohol. Then inject the medication into the shaft of the penis as directed by your doctor. (Most doctors who prescribe this medication educate the person well and will have the person perform the entire injection sequence in their office before allowing him to use the medication on his own.)

4. Dispose of the needle and syringe in an appropriate container and store the medication. On the side of the vial, mark the date the medication was first opened.

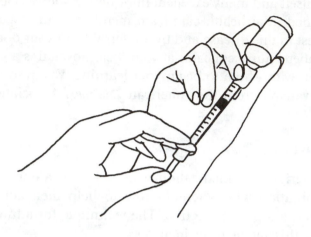

Drawing up injectable medication.

Intravenous

In many areas, home intravenous therapy is available. Most of the organizations providing this service are conscientious and cautious. Treatment with injectables should always include trained members of the health care team regardless of who actually injects the medications.

Know Your Service Provider

Here are a few tips on your relationship with providers of injectable products and services. These apply regardless of whether you or someone else will be administering the medications.

1. Expect a patient handbook that details:

   the services to be provided

   who will be paying the bill

   who will be training you and your alternate

   who will be making home visits and how often they will be made

2. You should receive written, illustrated directions that detail care of your injection site and device and precisely how the injectable medications are to be administered.

3. Get references for the business and check them out. This is not rude. It will help to establish your trust in the service provider.

4. If you will have to pay for the service and products, get a cost estimate. Injectable therapy can be extremely costly. Make sure you can afford this therapy alternative.

5. Make sure that care is provided around the clock and that you can always reach a person, not just a machine.

6. You should be provided with a written statement on each of your intravenous or central catheter medications telling their intent and other medication information you learned in Chapter 5.

Injectables Mean Special Caution is Necessary

Any time your bloodstream is accessed, there is a need for sterility. Otherwise, there is a high risk for infections.

Administering medications into the bloodstream cuts down on your body's chances to protect itself should there not be sterility. Home intravenous injection can be a safe and effective method of keeping you out of the hospital, but must be approached cautiously and systematically.

Training in Injection Techniques

Generally, your injectable training is begun in the hospital so you have an opportunity to practice the required techniques with round-the-clock professional support. These techniques include administration of the drug, clean up, storage of injectable medication, and ordering. You and a caregiver or backup person should receive both verbal and in-depth written and illustrated directions.

A safe alternative to in-hospital training can be home care teaching by a nurse or pharmacist. Most people develop more confidence when they are trained in the hospital *before* having to become responsible for the therapy themselves. Make your feelings on this topic known to your health care team members.

In review, medication-taking behavior can be broken down into a few steps that will help keep your medicine from ruling you. If you have further questions or need clarification, ask a member of your health care team.

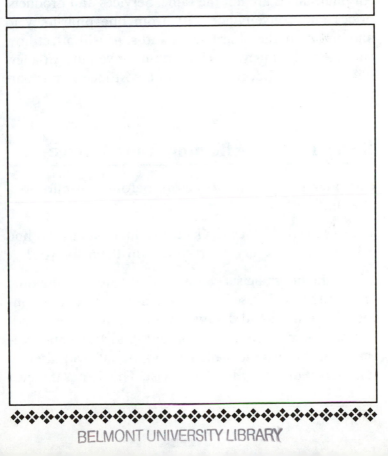

Chapter 10

Choosing a Pharmacy

Choosing a pharmacy is an important decision you make regarding your health care. This is especially true if you take medication for chronic conditions, take numerous prescriptions, or get medication from several prescribers. The benefit of a good pharmacist cannot be calculated in mere dollars and cents. By providing the medication along with the appropriate counseling, your pharmacist helps you use your health care dollars wisely. Counseling consists of an ongoing interaction between you and your pharmacist and results in safe and effective use of your medications.

All pharmacies are not the same. Services and products, prices and convenience vary from one pharmacy to another. Also, the pharmacists and staff will affect how you rate a pharmacy. It is important for you to tour a few pharmacies and decide which one best meets your particular needs.

Some Factors Affecting Your Choice

Consider the following factors before you choose a pharmacy.

1. Does the pharmacy stock the products you use? If not, will they make every effort to obtain them for you?

2. Are the pharmacists willing and able to take the time to discuss your prescription and nonprescription concerns? You need and deserve consultation on your medications. Some pharmacies permit clerks to hand prescriptions to customers and ring up the sale with little or no interaction with the pharmacist. This is not the best way to get your medications. Fortunately, pharmacists who routinely counsel people on medications are usually easy to identify. By watching the operation of the prescription area as it serves several people with their prescription needs, you will be able to see the degree of interaction between patients and pharmacists.

Sharing the information learned from years of training and practice is the most important part of what your pharmacist does for you. In some states, counseling on prescriptions by a pharmacist is actually mandated.

3. Is there adequate privacy to talk about sensitive matters? Topics like bladder control or vaginal infections can be awkward to discuss. A crowd of onlookers can make it uncomfortable.

4. Is the staff friendly and professional?

5. When you need advice on medications and self-medicating will you feel comfortable calling your pharmacist for information?

6. Is the staff eager to help you find the products you are looking for? Do they recognize and respond to special needs you may have? For example, if you have a hard time getting around because of breathing problems or arthritis, will they help you do your shopping, offer you a chair, or make sure aisles are uncluttered so you can navigate them?

7. Are the prices in line with those of other pharmacies in your area? Compare products you might be interested in buying. However, remember that special services such as delivery, special packaging, and insurance filing take time, and time is money. These added services and attention may be well worth the extra cost charged by the pharmacy.

8. Can you receive extra clinical services you might need like blood pressure monitoring, help with your blood glucose meter, a supply of wound treatment products, ostomy products, prostheses, special hosiery, braces and fittings, medical equipment, and intravenous therapy?

9. Is the location convenient? Can you gain access to the building easily? Is there parking nearby?

10. Will they file insurance forms for you or help you do it? Can you get periodic printouts of all your prescription purchases?

11. If you need delivery service, is it available?

Other factors may also affect your choice. The objective here is to get you started thinking about pharmacy selection in a systematic way.

Choosing a Single Pharmacy

Using one pharmacy to help you with your health care needs is better than using several. The world of medicine has become quite specialized and complex. You may have multiple prescribers ordering prescription and non-prescription medications.

1. Using a single pharmacy means that regardless of the source of your prescriptions, your pharmacy will have them all on record. Your pharmacist will be able to quickly and competently answer medication questions. New prescriptions will be filled only after your pharmacist has determined that there is no conflict with your current medications. Refills are monitored for compliance to help assure the desired outcome.

2. Another advantage of having one pharmacy is that the staff will get to know you. Then, if some change occurs in your physical appearance or skills, they will be likely to note it and help you decide if your prescriber should be notified.

3. In addition, the nonprescription purchases you make can be checked against the list of your prescription medications. This way you'll be less likely to buy products that interact adversely or duplicate each other. This will decrease your risks from multiple medications and will save you money.

4. It is even helpful for an entire family to patronize the same pharmacy.

Quality and Savings

Establishing a working relationship with your pharmacist is a way to improve your health, cut down on medical problems, and avoid the purchase of unnecessary products. While price is important, older people need pharmacy *services* more than any other group. If you aren't receiving the help you need, tell your pharmacist about it. If you don't get satisfaction, check to see if it is available elsewhere. If you choose a pharmacy care-fully, it is likely you will get both quality service and good prices.

Chapter 11

Filling and Refilling Prescriptions

❖❖❖❖❖❖❖❖❖❖❖❖❖❖❖❖❖❖❖❖❖❖❖❖❖❖❖❖

This chapter deals with the "nuts and bolts" of prescription filling and refilling. As you probably know, there are some tricks to getting it done quickly and painlessly. You will find the advantages and disadvantages of some alternative approaches to prescription filling. These include having the prescription called in by the doctor, taking the prescription to the pharmacy yourself, sending the prescription with another person, or mailing it to the pharmacy.

The pharmacist's role in filling your prescriptions is detailed from the initial review of your medication profile, generic substitution possibilities, and counseling on the proper use of the prescription. Prescription refills are discussed so you will know when they are suggested, permissible, or not allowed.

Filling a Prescription

There are a number of ways to approach filling a new prescription. Depending on the situation, some approaches will work more smoothly than others.

Four Options

1. You can have the prescription called in to the pharmacy by the prescriber or prescriber's nurse.

2. You can hand carry the prescription to your pharmacy.

3. You can send someone else to the pharmacy to get the prescription filled.

4. You can send the prescription to your pharmacy and request that it be mailed or delivered to you at home.

Pharmacist's Choice

With new prescriptions, an excellent choice is to have the prescriber call the prescription to your regular pharmacy. This way it will probably be filled when you arrive to pick it up. This approach is a good one for pharmacists because it gives them the chance to review your medication profile, resolve any concerns, and fill the prescription without a rush. With the prescription filled, your time in the pharmacy can be spent discussing the prescription with your pharmacist.

This is also the best approach when you are not feeling well and wish to avoid waiting in the pharmacy. It is also ideal for hospital discharge prescriptions. As a matter of fact, pharmacists encourage prescribers to phone in *all* discharge prescriptions. The prospect of a person waiting in the car or the pharmacy for medications on the way home from the hospital seems unpleasant and unnecessary.

When You Bring The Prescription With You

If you personally deliver the prescription to be filled, don't be in a hurry. You've probably been through the entire health care system by the time you get to the pharmacy. Now is the time to relax. Your pharmacist provides the last link in the chain that gets the right medication to you. This last step in resolving a health problem is an important one. You want everything to be checked and rechecked. Before the prescription is delivered to you for consultation, everything about the new medicine must be correct. Your pharmacist makes sure your medication, dose, and dosing schedule are appropriate for treating your condition. If it doesn't seem just right, inquiries are made. Occasionally, this may require more time than you were expecting to spend.

When Another Person Brings Your Prescription

This is not the best choice of ways to get your prescription filled. Because you know the answers to questions the pharmacist may have and your envoy probably doesn't, this method can sometimes end up taking extra time and telephone calls. If you must send someone else with your prescription, try to be available by telephone at that time.

Mailing the Prescription

This, too, is not an ideal way to have prescriptions filled. First, you are not available to answer the pharmacist's questions. Second, the pharmacist won't be there when you receive the prescription so you won't get all the information about the medication that you need. Save this method for a last resort. You get the product, but not all the services you need and deserve.

What the Pharmacist Does

In the business of filling prescriptions, much of what the pharmacist does may be unknown to you. Come to the pharmacists' side of the prescription counter so you can see how they serve you.

Review Of Your Medication Profile and History

As part of your prescription service, the pharmacist will:

1. Check for drug allergies.

2. Review your past and present medications
   a. to rule out duplications in therapy
   b. to identify potential drug interactions
   c. to be sure that your new medication is not just being used to treat preventable side effects from one of your other medications.

3. Consult with other members of the health care team if concerns or questions arise.

As you might imagine, these reviews take a few minutes. You deserve it.

Generic Substitution

If the prescription passes all of the checks against your medication profile or record, it will be filled. You will be asked if you wish a brand name product or a generic. In many cases, if you have prescription insurance, you will already have made this decision. Your insurance policy is where you will find the constraints on what products will be paid for. Your pharmacist attempts to keep up-to-date on the changes in insurance coverage for the companies most often seen in his or her area. It is helpful if you also read the insurance company updates on drug coverage so you know when you do and don't have a choice about generics.

If you have the option to choose between generic and brand medications, you will find the choice is not nearly as complex as it appears to be. When a manufacturer develops a new medication it is patented through the U.S. Government Patent Office. This gives the manufacturer of the new medication 17 years of exclusive marketing rights. Once the patent expires, other manufacturers may produce and market the drug under the generic name or some other brand name. The appropriate use of quality generic drug products can save you money while providing the medication therapy you need.

The Food and Drug Administration (FDA) establishes the standards that allow for a comparison of one manufacturer's drug product to another. This important process helps pharmacists determine whether one medication can be substituted for another. One FDA procedure tests the dissolution of the medication to see if it will dissolve reliably and be available for absorption into the body. Once it is dissolved, each generic medication must deliver roughly the same amount of active ingredient as the "standard" product. The generic can deliver 20 percent more or less than the "standard" product.

Twenty percent seems like a big variation, but it is not significant for most medications. Our bodies also vary a lot. Usually, product substitution causes no change in the therapy at all. There are some medications whose levels have to be closely monitored and controlled. With these medications, switching between one manufacturer's product and another can be risky. They may not deliver the same amount of active medication in the same time frame. Most pharmacists will not recommend substituting one brand for another in these cases.

Counseling

Once filled, the prescription container is labeled and the product is priced. You will be counseled on the correct use of the medication by your pharmacist. It is not always easy to learn all about each prescription the first time it is dispensed to you. Expect to learn part of the essential medication information each time the prescription is filled. Instructions may be written, verbal, or both. Be sure to let the pharmacist know if you have special communication needs. Finally, a clerk will ring up the sale.

Refills

Don't wait until you are out of medication to decide to get a refill. Lots of things can keep you from receiving a refill as fast as you wish. For example, the prescriber will have to be contacted if the prescription has expired or there are no refills left. If the prescriber is not in the office that day, then the refill will wait a day. Generally, pharmacists can advance you a few tablets of a maintenance medication, but not always. Try to order a prescription refill about 5 days before you will run out.

When The Prescription Label Says No Refills

Before calling or going to the pharmacy, check the refill status of your medication. The number of remaining refills should appear on the prescription label. If no refills are permitted, action must be taken by someone. It may be you or it may be adequate for your pharmacist to call the doctor's office. A few things to consider before you decide who should make the phone call are:

1. Do you know the prescriber's intent for giving you the medication?

2. Were you to continue taking the medication?

3. Were you to be seen by the prescriber to check your progress before refilling the prescription?

4. What was the date of your last appointment? Maybe it's time for your routine checkup.

Your regular pharmacist will have a good idea from this information as to whether the prescriber will issue refills without your being seen or at least talked with.

Regardless of who calls the prescriber, your medical records will probably have to be pulled from the files and sent to your prescriber. He or she will then have to take time to review your chart and decide on a course of action. This can take time.

The Routine Refill

If you are on a maintenance medication, you will have to routinely refill the prescription. This is not an unimportant task. Complying with long term medication therapy can make a significant difference in how well your condition is treated or controlled. To help monitor compliance, pharmacists' records allow them to assess whether you are refilling your prescription at the correct intervals. If you are not, the pharmacist may question you about it. Perhaps the dose has changed or you are having trouble remembering to take it. In the practice of pharmacy, it is not enough to just sell medications. The outcome of your therapy and your ultimate well-being are what is monitored.

A Lifetime Supply

There is often some misunderstanding about the issue of refills on lifetime medications. People like to get the maximum number of refills from their prescribers. As much as possible, prescribers try to accommodate the people they serve. But they keep the person's best interest in mind by limiting refills. At first glance, this might seem obstructive, but further examination reveals solid reasons for it.

Health care teams working with state legislatures have developed regulations regarding refills. Restrictions have been created for a number of reasons. First, treatment may change. Second, pharmaceutical technology has been creating more and better medication that may be preferable to the ones you currently take. Third, people and their bodies change. Some changes that you might experience can necessitate alterations to medication therapy. These include:

1. Major weight gain or loss,

2. Change of habits, especially if you quit smoking or change the amount of alcohol you drink,

3. Functional changes like inability to walk that may result in reduced muscle mass,

4. Newly diagnosed conditions such as changes in kidney or liver functions,

5. Addition of new medications or changes in other aspects of your drug regimen,

6. Normal aging.

The regulations requiring patients to be reevaluated on a regular basis before renewing prescriptions are truly consumer oriented and protective.

Helpful Hints

1. If your prescriber changes the directions for one of your prescriptions, have him or her write a new prescription that reflects the current directions. This way your compliance can be monitored, your medication records will show what is currently ordered, and insurance will be appeased.

2. If you change prescribers, for example, if your doctor retires or moves away, get new prescriptions from your

new doctor as soon as possible. In some states, prescriptions or their refills are not valid once the relationship between you and the prescriber ceases.

Time-Consuming Snags in Prescription Filling

As with any of life's activities, there are some things that can impede progress in prescription filling. Here are a few irritations you can help avoid.

1. *No one can identify the prescriber's name.* This happens frequently. Legally, the prescriber's name must appear on your prescription label. Often the unidentified doctor is a specialist the person doesn't know well. Sometimes it is a practitioner covering for the person's regular doctor in his or her absence. Either way, it can take time to track down this person. Prevent this delay by looking over the prescription before you leave the doctor's office or hospital. Be sure the prescriber prints his or her name below the signature on all your orders and prescriptions. This will also help you if you need to contact the prescriber with questions or problems regarding your condition, and it will help your pharmacist fill your prescription.

2. *The prescriber refuses to make a long-distance call to your pharmacy.* The remedy for this potential snag is to get the prescriber's full name, phone number and how long he or she can be reached at that phone number. Then call your pharmacy and explain the situation. Pharmacists will usually make the call themselves.

3. *You are going to a new pharmacy.* Be prepared to give all vital information when the prescription is first presented. This includes name; address; phone; birthdate; insurance; allergies; other ongoing therapy; and special considerations like duplicate receipts, delivery, or no safety caps. Before leaving the pharmacy, ask for a pharmacy business card. Remember that the pharmacy name, address, and phone number are also on every prescription label.

Filling and refilling your prescriptions are important parts of safe and effective medication therapy. Since there are many other facets of medication therapy, it is good to keep each of them as simple as possible. By mastering this important part of independent medication management, you can improve the outcome of your therapy, which will in turn improve your health and save you money.

Chapter 12

Safety and
Nonsafety Caps

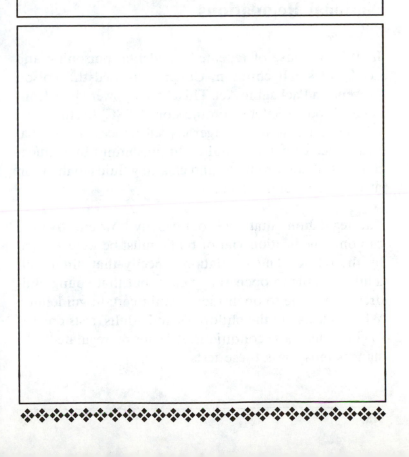

Many consumers are annoyed by the safety caps that come on prescription vials and bottles. They wonder why these inconvenient and annoying caps are being used. The answer comes from the Federal Poison Prevention Packaging Act of 1970. This chapter will give you some history of poison prevention packaging, also known as child resistant packaging or safety caps. You will see exactly what the regulations expect from safety caps. Included are some tips for opening the most difficult of caps and advice on some things to avoid.

National Regulations

In 1970, because of repeated accidental poisoning and deaths of small children, Congress passed the Poison Prevention Packaging Act. This Act empowered the Consumer Product Safety Commission (CPSC) to study and regulate packages of dangerous substances. Their goal was to decrease accidental child poisonings by medication, petroleum products, and cleaning fluids to mention just a few potential hazards.

The regulations that spell out exactly how effective the cap on a medication vial or bottle must be were created by the CPSC. The regulations specify that almost all adults be able to open safety caps, but that young children be unable to open them within certain guidelines. What follows are the children's and adults' tests created to guarantee these conditions. All caps on regulated substances must pass these tests.

The Children's Test

The capped package, either a vial or bottle, is given to 200 children age 42 to 51 months (roughly 3½ to 4¼ years). The children are tested in pairs. Each child is handed a closed package and asked to open it. This part of the test is 5 minutes long. If the child fails to open the package, the method of opening is demonstrated *without* verbal instruction. The child is then given another 5 minutes to open the package. The regulations specify that for the cap to pass the test, no more than 15 percent of the children can open the packages without the demonstration and that no more than 20 percent of children can get them open in the total 10 minutes.

The Adults' Test

The other test is to see if adults 18 to 45 years old with no obvious handicaps, and 70 percent of whom are female, can open the packages. The adults are tested individually rather than in pairs. The adults get only printed material explaining the mechanism of the cap. They are given 5 minutes to open and close the package. The regulations specify that for the cap to pass the test, 90 percent of the adults must be able to open and close the package in 5 minutes.

Complications

All the caps are tested in well people under age 46. Elderly people who have to contend with the same caps may not be as strong or flexible or see as well as the younger adults. The good news, however, is that some studies show many elderly people can do just as well as their younger counterparts.

One study on skills of elderly patients related to opening and closing prescription vials disclosed that while many of the people say the safety caps are difficult and a nuisance, the vast majority of these people can open and close the vials within 1 minute. This study group was mainly men who may have a lower incidence of severe arthritis than women. People with arthritis or other musculoskeletal conditions might find the task more difficult. The results of other studies vary depending on the safety cap chosen, the disability of the people opening the caps, and the diameter of the vials used.

Tricks for Opening Various Caps

People with difficulty opening the various safety caps can learn some tricks that may make the task easier. Because safety caps come in many types, you will eventually encounter one that gives you trouble. Your skills and general abilities may vary and these tricks can be helpful when you are having a rough day. Knowing the easy way to work with safety caps will also help you resist the temptation to store your medications in less safe containers. One general tip is this: Before leaving your pharmacy, check to be sure the caps are familiar to you. If they are not, ask your pharmacist to demonstrate how to open and close the medication containers.

Press Down and Turn Caps

To get caps off that are labeled "Press Down and Turn," place the vial on a countertop about hip high. If grip strength is a problem, hold the vial upright on a damp sponge. This will keep it in one place. Using the ball of your hand (right by your thumb), press on the cap. Turn your entire torso counterclockwise. This eliminates the need to twist your wrist. After the twist, the cap will pull right off. The illustration below shows one such vial and cap.

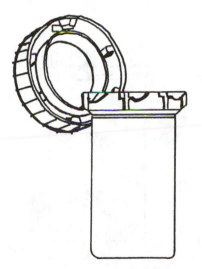

"Press down and turn" cap and vial.

Matching Arrows

If you get a product with the kind of closure that requires lining up two arrows, try this. First, line up the arrows or have someone do it for you. Next, draw a dark line through the arrows with a magic marker to show how the vial looks when it is aligned for opening. Now your cap is ready. To open, turn the cap until the two halves of the line are matched up. Then, lift the cap. When replacing the cap, again match up the lines, push the cap down, and turn it slightly. Turning the cap will seal it so the contents are safe and don't fall out. Be sure you recap the vial each time you open it. The illustration below details the closure of this vial.

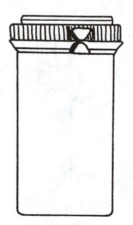

Safety cap requiring alignment of arrows on the cap and the vial.

Large Diameter Vials

If you always seem to have problems getting your prescription caps off, ask the pharmacist to package your prescriptions in a larger diameter vial than you normally get. It is easier to get a grip on a larger vial.

The Combination Cap

These plastic caps look something like an elevated bowl. The base of the bowl is the nonsafety portion and the bowl itself is the safety part. These caps can be screwed onto the prescription vial to yield a nonsafety closure. If the other end of the cap is screwed onto the vial it makes a safety closure. The safety portion of the cap has a tab that must be pressed in order for the cap to twist off. The illustration below shows this type of vial and cap.

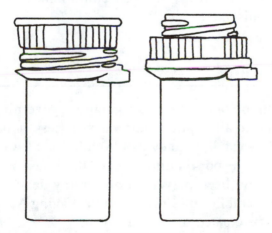

Dual purpose safety/nonsafety cap and vial.

Nonsafety Caps

Finally, if you have tried every approach for opening safety caps without success, ask to receive nonsafety caps on your prescription containers. This is a last resort for most people. If you use nonsafety caps on your medication, you should store it out of sight and in a locked cabinet.

Precautions

Do not leave a cap off or partially off medication containers. Even if you store the medication on a high shelf or hidden in a drawer, this is not safe storage. It may jeopardize other people, and it exposes your medications to improper storage conditions. Don't transfer your medications from one container to another unless you also transfer the label. Taking medication from unlabeled or incorrectly labeled containers can lead to harmful mistakes.

Conclusion

The intention of the law and regulations governing safety closures is to allow adults fairly easy access while assuring that if you take your eyes off a child for a few minutes, he or she won't poison him- or herself. Thousands of poisonings have been prevented and many deaths averted by the Federal Poison Prevention Packaging Act and the safety caps created as a result of it.

Chapter 13

Medication Costs

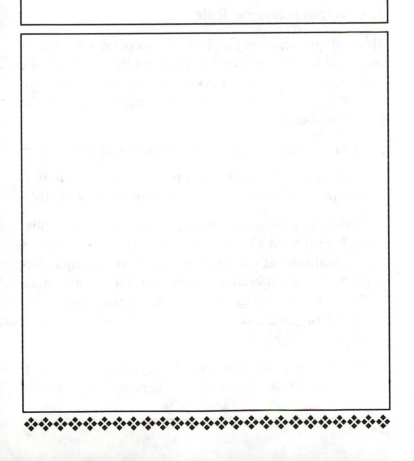

The cost of medication therapy is a concern to us all. This chapter will explain why medication costs what it does and what you can do to lessen these costs. Some inappropriate ways of saving money are discussed along with what to do when you see your resources running out.

Reasons That Medication Costs Are High

The Manufacturer's Role

Although prescription medications make up a small portion of all health care costs, they are visible to the public and often paid for out of pocket. Currently, the bulk of what you pay is product cost. It is determined by the drug manufacturer.

Some of the factors that contribute to product costs are:

1. Protection of the market by a patent so the drug manufacturer can recoup research and development costs.

2. Marketing strategies including such practices as raising the price on a medication when the patent expires and multi-tiered pricing, which means the manufacturer charges different amounts to different customers. This pricing strategy differs from what is allowed by the federal government for producers of other goods in the United States.

3. Advertising costs that include sales representatives, trinkets with the drug logo on them, mailings, media

advertising, and giving "free" samples of medications to doctors.

4. Contributions to the medical health field. These include seminars, publications, and grants to professionals and organizations for meetings and research.

5. Stockholder dividends.

6. The presence of little competition between manufacturers of similar medications. This may mean that treatment with a particular type of medication will cost essentially the same regardless of which brand is ordered.

7. The ability of manufacturers to create their own competition by introducing generics that are then marketed against the name brand products owned by the same company.

The Pharmacist's Role

A dispensing fee or markup is added to the cost of the product by the pharmacist. This dispensing fee or markup covers the pharmacy's cost of doing business and allows the owner to make a profit. These costs will vary by pharmacy location, the cost of the medication, and services rendered. Over the last 8 to 10 years, pharmacists' reimbursement independent from product costs has essentially remained the same or decreased. In part, this is a result of increased competition and efficiency of operation.

Presently, pharmacists don't have a separate charge for the expense of time spent on phone calls, medication profile review to detect interactions or duplications, or for counseling. Special packaging like "bingo" cards that contain all the medication for one dosing time or unit dose, where the medicine is packaged and labeled in single doses may cost extra.

Controlling Costs

Getting your money's worth is not impossible. Here are some suggestions that may save you money.

1. *The main thing you can do is use your medications wisely.* This means taking them as directed for the period specified by your prescriber. It also means using teamwork to decide on dosing changes. Keeping your health care team informed about your progress, including your frustrations, is important in getting the desired outcome of therapy at the lowest possible cost.

2. *Use of generic substitutes, if appropriate, can save you money.* Many quality generic products are available and approved by the FDA as equivalent to the brand medication. Most states allow for substitution of these generics. There are some prescriptions for which pharmacists would not substitute or use a generic. Trust your pharmacist to help you make this choice. However, you should keep track of your progress and side effects. It is possible to react slightly differently even to an approved generic brand. For example, the original brand or the generic brand might dissolve slightly faster than the other. It is possible for this to result in a side effect such as a feeling of fullness, a headache, or whatever other side effects the medication is known for.

3. *Seek a good product at a reasonable price and stick with it.* There is little benefit from jumping around from one brand to another.

4. *Keeping good records can help save you money.* Both people and their prescribers move around the country more than ever before. New prescribers may inadvertently choose to prescribe a medication that didn't work for you in the past. These days, it helps if your records show what medications have been tried and what the outcome of their use was. See Chapter 7, Keeping A Medication Diary.

5. *Ask your doctor what the goal of therapy is and whether you must continue to take the medication once the goal is met.* For example, if you take a medicine for stomach ulcers and the ulcer is healed, do you have to continue the medication? Particularly with skin disorders, people are not sure what to do once they have reached their goal. By stopping medication at the appropriate time, you save money and are not exposed to medication for longer than needed.

6. *If the medication is intended to be taken for a long time, you can ask if the price per unit decreases if you buy larger quantities.* Perhaps it is less expensive if you buy 30 tablets rather than 15 tablets at a time. This kind of price reduction is possible because it saves the pharmacist from having to go through all the steps of refilling your prescription an extra time. When the special price is possible, it can be beneficial for you.

7. *Don't buy huge quantities of medications.* They will be wasted if your regimen changes or if temperature and humidity affects them. A 1- or 2-month supply of your routine medications should be plenty. This keeps you from having to go to the pharmacy when the weather is terrible, but doesn't load you down with possibly danger-ous or useless medications. It also leaves some money in your pocket to use until the next refill is needed.

8. *Newer medications are almost always more expensive than medications that have been on the market for a while.* Ask your doctor to check with your pharmacist to see if the other alternatives for treating your condition are less expensive.

What to Do if You Can't Afford Your Medication

Look for solutions to financial problems before your situation becomes desperate. Medication is a necessity like lights, water, housing, and food. Do not wait until you have no money to pay for these things before you start looking for assistance. Experience has shown that county social agencies may be the fastest to respond to an impending financial crisis. You may want to contact them if you need help. Another solution is to let someone on your health care team know your difficulties. There may be something they can do to provide help or direct you to a source of help. They may have experience in solving problems like yours and will be glad to help you if they can.

Inappropriate Ways to Try to Save Money

You may be tempted to try to make medication last longer or cost less. Most of the time you will not benefit by cutting corners. At the very least, your therapy will be compromised. Some examples that illustrate inappropriate ways to adjust medication therapy are:

1. Being lured by a well-meaning friend's offer to share medication. This is an unsafe practice. Only your doctor or pharmacist should dispense medications to you.

2. Adjusting your dosing schedule to try to make medication last longer. Your doctor prescribed what he or she believes is the minimum effective dose to treat your condition. Taking less than the prescribed amount may mean that your condition will not be adequately treated.

3. Discontinuing any of your medications for any reason without talking to your doctor and pharmacist. Remember *you* are part of a health care team.

   There are many ways people attempt to stretch their medication, but what these attempts really do is to inadequately treat the medical condition. Improper treatment can result in the need for more or revised therapy or even in the need for hospitalization.

Long-Term Goals in Cost Control

Political action is one powerful tool for achieving long-term goals in health care. Elderly people have shown they can use their political clout as well as any group in the United States. In a grassroots approach, you can join friends in learning about the issues in health care costs. Expressing your carefully thought-out opinions on these issues is both a right and responsibility. You can help to identify the most pressing health care problems and suggest solutions to them.

Chapter 14

Seeing Your Doctor

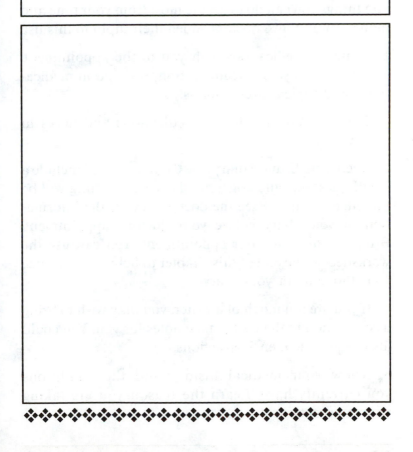

In the not-so-distant past, our only responsibilities for a doctor's appointment were to show up clean and on time. Things have changed. As we became partners in our health care, we accepted the duty to be more knowledge-able and prepared when we meet with our doctors.

Preparing for the Appointment

In anticipation of a doctor's appointment, there are certain things you can do to get the most from your time and money. Twenty-two doctors added their input to this list.

1. Bring *all* medications with you to the appointment. This includes eye medications, nonprescription medications, and topical preparations.

2. Carry an updated list of medications and doses in your wallet.

3. Keep a medication diary (see Chapter 7) and include a list of questions and concerns. This way nothing will be forgotten when you see the doctor. Review the information in your diary before your doctor's appointment. Bring the diary to your appointment. You can use the worksheet at the end of this chapter to help you organize your thoughts in your diary.

4. If you are not much of a writer, you may wish to bring a companion to the visit to take notes for you. You could also request written instructions.

5. Know your medical history and the conditions you currently have. Learn the reason you are taking your medications.

6. Know your medication allergies.

7. If you plan to arm yourself with information you have read about your medications and medical conditions, use appropriate references. There are many drug reference books available. Some like the *United States Pharmacopoeia Dispensing Information* and *Advice for the Patient* are unbiased comprehensive sources of information for the layperson. Layperson refers here to a person who is not trained as a chemist, physician, or pharmacologist. Your pharmacist can provide you with copies of the information about your specific medications from the *USP-DI*. As an alternative, you could purchase the books, *About Your Medications* or *The Pill Book*. Some of the books that are widely available are less helpful for you because they are written for audiences with more science training than the average person has. Books specifically written for health care professionals are not adequate resources for most people.

8. Plan to arrive in plenty of time so you aren't anxious about keeping the appointment. If you are relying on someone else for a ride home, try to make the plans flexible so you won't have to rush around to get out of the office so as not to inconvenience your driver.

9. If you use glasses or a hearing aid, wear them.

10. Once you have established the purpose of the visit try to stick to it. Use the information you have prepared with the help of the worksheet and information in your medication diary.

What to Do During Your Appointment with the Doctor

1. Know exactly how you are taking your medication. When asked, be honest about how you are taking it. Only accurate information is useful.

2. If you suspect adverse effects from your medication, document the details such as what occurred and when. Report these to the doctor before stopping the therapy.

3. Plan to write down new instructions. You will know and remember exactly what transpired if you write down important information *during* the appointment. Include the prescriber's name, new instructions, and opinions voiced to you. Read these back to the staff to be sure you have them right. If anyone acts impatient remind them that this will probably save them a phone call and pulling up your medical record later. You don't need to say it, but remind yourself that this is a service that you have a right to and are paying for. You have fulfilled your obligation by coming prepared for the visit.

4. Make sure you can see and hear in the examining room. Tell the staff if you are having trouble.

5. Stay calm. You'll be more apt to remember things.

6. Don't withhold your concerns; air them. That way you will be participating in the decisions being made. You will have confidence in the therapy decided on because you were part of the process.

Changes since your last appointment are important to report. They give your doctor important information about your health and the therapy you receive.

7. As part of the visit, ask about nondrug alternatives. Dietary changes and life-style adjustments can often be used to combat medical conditions. Evaluate these non-drug suggestions with your prescriber to determine if they would be appropriate. If not, at least you are informed about these options. Keep an open mind toward them.

8. Ask both prescriber and dispenser about side effects that may occur from proposed medication. Will they go away? Are they dangerous? Will they be short-lived? Will they last while therapy continues? Should they be tolerated as being less noxious than the condition being treated? Are the risks greater from taking or omitting the medication?

What to Expect from Your Doctor's Visit

Don't expect to come away with a prescription at every visit. A prescription may be unnecessary. Further, though you have been told that you may have to take a medication "for the rest of your life," don't expect to get a prescription with infinite refills on it. Your prescriber has more respect for you than to assume nothing will change or that no monitoring is necessary.

In most states, a year or 15 months is the maximum any prescription can be filled. As mentioned previously in Chapter 11, laws governing this were created to be sure you are monitored for the correctness of diagnosis, medication, dose, and development of side effects or other conditions that could affect therapy. Just as our external appearance changes as we age, our internal needs also change.

Is Satisfaction Possible?

What will satisfy you as far as outcome of therapy? Can it be achieved by the suggested therapy? By any therapy? What's the best outcome to be expected? Go ahead and discuss these questions with your doctor or nurse. No one is better qualified than they are to answer them.

Chapter 14 Worksheet

Preparing for a Doctor's Appointment

Your name:

Today's date:

Main reason for Doctor visit and main health complaint:

Current medications, dose, and dosing schedule of each:

Reason these medications are being taken:

Problems with medication:

New prescriptions:

Condition to be treated:

Name of new medication:

How it should be taken:

For how long should it be taken:

Expected outcome:

Any other medication changes made:

Questions: Answers:

When to return to doctor:

Chapter 15

Coping with Emergencies

This chapter presents information on recognizing and coping with emergencies. Planning is the key to successfully weathering an emergency. Your doctor, the rest of your health team, and you have a role in knowing what to do in a crisis.

What Your Doctor Suggests

It is good to know in advance what you should do if a situation becomes serious. It is doubtful you will always know how to react, but you can reassure yourself by asking some basic questions of your doctor beforehand.

Ask specifically:

1. Under what circumstances should you call the doctor?

2. Under what circumstances should you go straight to an emergency room?

Write down the answers your doctor gives in your medication diary. This will help you learn the answers and will give you a chance to review the information if you are in doubt.

Answers from Other Members of Your Health Care Team

You may also want to discuss emergencies with other members of your health care team who are actively involved with your care including the nurse, pharmacist, or occupational therapist. Ask for ideas on both dealing with and preventing crises.

Find out:

1. What special instructions or suggestions each of these individuals have for you. For example, a pharmacist might remind you to post a conspicuous note in your home telling where your medications and medication diary are stored. An occupational therapist might remind you to change the batteries in your smoke alarm and learn how to get to the exits in your home.

2. Which team member to contact in any particular situation.

3. What information you should gather about your condition in order for the team to help you make crisis decisions.

Again, *write* down any instructions they provide in your medication diary.

What You Can Do

You can see that your role in planning is to gather, organize and preserve information. It's okay to get a little carried away with this task. Cover all the bases. Make a list of all the information sources you might ever use. Highlight the main ones. This could include your doctor's name and office phone number, county social worker, County Commission on Aging, police, rescue squad, State Department of Aging, religious connections, and names of friends. Decide now when you'd want to use these numbers. Post them by the phone.

Investigate the advantages of creating a Durable Power of Attorney for Health Care. This tool allows your opinion to be considered in your health care even if you are unable to express it in an emergency. Your doctor, social services agency, and local Department of Aging are good sources of information on this document.

What a Pharmacist Suggests

About Your Medications

1. Having your medications listed accurately in an easy-to-find place can help others care for you properly in an emergency. In some states, emergency rescue personnel are not allowed to look through your wallet. This means a wallet medication list won't help you unless you are able to hand it to them.

2. Keep your list up-to-date. Outdated information is nearly as bad as none at all. Pick a day to routinely update your medication list. For example, on the day of the change to and from daylight savings time, get out your lists and make sure they are current.

Information Systems

There are numerous ways to keep medication information available for your health care team in the event of an emergency.

The Vial of Life is one method of providing health information. You keep an updated medication list in a vial in the refrigerator. You apply a decal to your main door stating that you have a Vial of Life. If you are at home when the emergency arises, vital health information is available immediately. You can make your own version of this method if you are unable to purchase this product.

Another approach is a medical information bracelet or necklace. This has the advantage of being with you at all times. Some companies provide a 24-hour telephone number on the medallion for health care personnel to call and obtain information. You must update the company about changes in your therapies or allergy status. Medallions with your health conditions on them are obviously not as informative, but certainly better than no information.

Another approach is to tape a note on your phone or the inside of your door that tells where you keep your medications and medication diary.

Many other systems are available. Check with senior citizen programs in your local area, pharmacies, and physicians to see what they recommend. Regardless of the system you choose, remember that you must keep the information up to date for it to really be of assistance.

Trust Your Instincts

If you believe something is seriously wrong, you are probably right. For example, if the pain you are having is somehow different than anything you've had before, call for help. You may want to call the rescue squad or ambulance before making any other calls. This is true especially if you are confident you need emergency medical services. Your next call may be to a friend. It can be reassuring to have a friend come over to comfort you in a frightening situation. Calling a friend first may be important if you need advice from a person you trust.

Advanced planning can help you face emergencies so that you can expect the best possible outcome. Planning with the input of your health care team members is both smart and is one way to make emergencies less frightening.

Chapter 16

Hospitalization

A planned hospitalization such as for hernia repair or hip replacement can be handled like a routine doctor's appointment. Use the items mentioned in Chapter 14, Seeing Your Doctor, to help you organize your goals and questions. Write them in your medication diary. Make sure you take it with you along with an up-to-date list of your current medication regimen.

Unplanned Hospitalization

Unplanned hospital stays can be quite stressful. They show us all the frailties of our systems. From bringing in newspaper to paying the monthly bills, we see just how many activities are involved in our daily lives. Dealing with these things from a hospital bed can be an ordeal. You can alleviate some stress by being well organized in advance. Using the tips in Chapter 15, Coping With Emergencies, can make things go more smoothly for you. Your goal is to make your medication routine as clear and straightforward as possible so you will receive the appropriate care.

Chapter 5, Learning About Your Medications, taught that the first thing you should learn about your medication is what it is for. In an emergency, you will be more likely to remember your diagnosis accurately than to remember the precise name of your medications. Though it is incomplete, health care providers will find it more useful to know you take medicine for high blood pressure than to hear you are taking some medication that starts with an "h." Obviously the more correct and complete the information you provide, the better.

Opportunities to Learn While in the Hospital

Hospitals keep complete records of every dose of every medication you receive or is ordered for you. In most cases, medications will be administered to you by nursing or pharmacy staff. These days, however, there are opportunities for you to administer your own medications while in hospital. Some hospitals have self-administration medication programs (SAMPs) for patients on rheumatology (arthritis), geriatric, or psychiatric services. These programs are designed for people with chronic conditions and multiple medications. Being in a SAMP allows you to get control of a cumbersome medication regimen and become comfortable with any changes in it. In general, the length of stays in the hospital are decreasing so you may be discharged before you can be enrolled in a SAMP. If you believe you would benefit by SAMP, let your nurse and doctor know early.

Discharge Plans

Discharge can be one of the most confusing parts of hospital care. You will no doubt be anxious to get home, but you will need to stay as relaxed as possible because there is much to be done for you. Discharge may be a time when you will need to get some assistance. If you need to, get a friend or relative to be present at your discharge teaching. You may want that person to make notes for you on information you receive that day. A discharge checklist is included in this chapter to help you organize information.

Elderly people are often more debilitated by hospital stays than younger people and may have more difficulty assimilating new information presented before discharge. Most elderly people will learn perfectly well provided the information is repeated and reinforced. It appears that elderly people are often being discharged before they are well and "road worthy" because it's expensive to keep them in the hospital. Studies are now demonstrating that little is saved by this practice as hospital readmission and nursing home admission are more likely if someone is sent home from the hospital before he or she is ready to care for him- or herself.

To avoid the cycle of going home from the hospital, failing to thrive, and being rehospitalized, get some help at home for a week or more following hospital discharge. You need someone to help with some of the daily chores and with adapting to your new medication regimen. Most hospitals have social workers or discharge planners who can help to arrange for assistance in your home.

Items To Remember

1. *Discharge medication orders are often written at the last minute.* As a result, you may have to go to a pharmacy and wait while these prescriptions are filled. Try to get the prescriber to call the prescriptions to your pharmacy. They can be filled and ready when you arrive.

2. *If part of your medications have been discontinued, make a list of the ones to be discontinued so you can destroy them when you get home.*

3. *Be aware of how many doses of your medications you have taken on the day of hospital discharge.* Find out how many doses remain for that day. The excitement of going home may tire you. While you are still fresh and rested in the hospital, calculate your medication schedule for the rest of the day and the following day. Write it down in your medication diary.

4. *Just because you have been released from the hospital, don't expect everything to be instantly back to normal.* You have many things to learn about your new health conditions and the medications that treat them. You may need time to recover physically.

Hospital Discharge Checklist

Your Name:

Name of Hospital:

Discharge Date:

Caregiver's Name: Your Doctors' Names:

Conditions for which you were treated in this admission:

New Medication Regimen:
medication name   condition treated   strength   dose   schedule

What previous medication should be discontinued and discarded?

Medication schedule for DAY OF DISCHARGE:
medication name   strength   dose   time to take dose

If these symptoms occur, contact:
name   phone

Symptoms to watch for:

See Dr. _____ at _____A.M. P.M.

    on _____ , 199__

Chapter 17

Being a Caregiver

In this book, *caregiver* refers to someone who assists an elderly person with personal matters. Caregiver includes spouses, other relatives, and people who volunteer or are paid to help with the activities of daily living such as grocery shopping, housekeeping, or medication management. This chapter addresses some of the issues related to being a caregiver responsible for helping another person with medications. It focuses on why you would want to help a person with medication, to what degree you might decide to be involved, and for how long. It also discusses how to decide when *not* to get involved. Suggestions on how to organize your caregiver duties and some steps to take to protect yourself from accusations of improper behavior are included.

Why You Get Involved

The most obvious answer is that you care about someone, their health, and their independence. The need to intercede in the management of another person's medications can begin in response to a crisis or can occur as the result of gradual changes. The crisis could be a serious infection or other acute illness that causes confusion and an inability to get around the house to perform normal activities. Gradual changes could include the increasing inability to do tasks that used to be routine because of worsening arthritis or visual impairment. These changes may be due to aging or to the progression of an illness.

Before You Become the Caregiver

Get as many facts about the person's situation as you can. Success may require thought and planning before you approach the person who needs assistance. The situation will require good communication once you and the person begin to talk and work together.

Ask the Right Questions

To determine what the situation really is, you'll have to ask the right questions and help the person understand that finding solutions is the reason behind those questions. Interviewing is an art. If questions are not worded appropriately, you may not find out what you really want to know. Here is one tip that may make it easier for the person to tell you what you want to know. Ask questions that require an explanation and not just a yes or no answer. For example, you want to find out whether the person can read the label on a prescription container. You will get more useful information by asking, "Will you please read this label for me?" rather than saying, "Can you read this label?" In the first case, you will see and hear a demonstration of the skill. In the second, you'll probably get a one word answer that doesn't enlighten you much and that may actually be misleading.

Body Language

It is said that 60 percent of what we communicate is done nonverbally. Be aware of your own nonverbal cues. This goes to the issue of body language. Even if you think you know the answers to your questions, don't show it on your face or with your body language. Let the person tell you his or her version of the situation. The truth as he or she sees it may help you both find solutions to the problems faced.

Also watch the other person's body language. Does he or she seem particularly uncomfortable with a topic? Sometimes you'll be able to tell when to ask more about a topic because of what the person does not say out loud.

Tips for Communicating Successfully

Other communication tips include always being sure the person has clean eye glasses, if they wear glasses, when the two of you interact. Likewise, people with hearing aids should wear them and have functioning batteries. Eliminate background noises and distractions. Even with the sound turned down a television is a distraction. Turn on the lights in the room. Don't stand behind a person in a wheelchair and try to carry on a conversation. Face the person when either of you speaks. If the person sits, you sit, and if he or she stands, you stand. It is important to talk with each other at the same level.

Be Direct

Most important, decide what it is that you need to know. Then, ask the questions that will get you the information you are looking for. Beating around the bush will only confuse and frustrate both of you.

Helping the Other Person Solve Problems

Once you have answers to your questions you need to decide if the problems you face as a caregiver are simple or complex and permanent or reversible. Here are several examples of problems you may encounter as you talk with the person. They may turn out to have either simple or complex solutions.

1. The person who has always managed the checkbook is suddenly unable to balance it and write checks for the purchase of goods including medications. Possible explanations of this new disability include a new or worsened visual problem or some intellectual decline.

2. The person routinely runs out of medicine or admits to forgetting to refill prescriptions. This could indicate concern brought on by some disturbing report in the media about medications. It could be an attempt to save money. Or, it could signal advancing memory loss.

3. The person is using more OTC products than before to medicate vague new symptoms. It is possible that this means nothing more than that the person has some passing malady like the flu, a cold, or indigestion. Increased use of OTC products could also be a sign of increased prescription medication side effects or the onset of a new undiagnosed condition.

Your conversations with the person must be geared to sort out the possible reasons for a problem. When the problem appears to be a result of easily explained and remedied difficulties, you may be able to help by suggesting appropriate solutions. Some simple solutions to functional impairments include improving vision or hearing

to allow him or her to read prescription labels or to telephone refills to the pharmacy. Maybe a new prescription
for glasses, better in-home lighting, or cataract surgery can
resolve the problem. Sometimes ear wax removal will
dramatically improve hearing. Refill inconsistencies may
be explained by a lack of transportation to the pharmacy
to obtain refills. Solutions, like the problems they address,
may be simple or complex and short- or long-term.

Respect the Person's Rights

Always try to find solutions that maintain the person's
identity and independence. It is important to keep in
mind that a person's self-esteem may be eroded by making him or her unnecessarily dependent. Remember that
with a little time and encouragement, many tasks can be
accomplished by the person without your intervention.
Indeed, you may be able to help without daily involvement. If this is not possible, if it seems like a dramatic
intervention is necessary, you will have laid the proper
foundation. The intervention you agree to must be within
your skills, obligations, and rights as a caregiver.

Assess Your Position

There are many things to consider as you look toward a
future of involvement in another person's medication
care. Following is a list of some important questions to
ask *yourself* and the other people involved.

1. How did you get involved? Was it your choice? The person's choice? Or their family's request? The answer to these questions will influence both your and the person's sentiments about any relationship between the two of you.

2. Why did the person want *you* to manage the medication? There are probably obvious and hidden reasons.

3. What is your relationship to the person? Do you feel good about it? If not, why not? It's going to be hard to establish a working system if there are emotional barriers involved.

4. Who is qualified to take on this task? You? No single person? Is a more protective arrangement needed like protected housing or nursing home care?

5. Are you willing and able to learn new information and adapt to new circumstances? Being a caregiver will probably require it.

6. Even if you are qualified, can you fulfill the role? For example, if you had to be at the person's home every day but he or she lives far from you and you don't drive, could you work it out? Would you need to be able to lift more weight than you think you can? Consider everything.

7. Who do you think *should* be providing the care? What does the person think about this?

8. What does the job entail? You wouldn't take any other job without some idea of the tasks you'd be doing. Caregiving is not an exception. Get a "job descrip-

tion" that details what needs to be done, in what time frame and for how long a period of time. You may find that help is needed not only with medications but also with other activities of daily living. In this case, you should decide if you want and are able to do them. Or perhaps there are agencies or other people that can take care of those matters.

9. What is the expected duration of your help? Is the need temporary such as following surgery, or is it expected to be long-term as in the irreversible changes of dementia?

10. What will happen if you can't or won't continue to provide the care?

11. What is your motivation for getting involved as a medication caregiver? Be sure the other person is at the center of your motivation to help. Your rewards may be few.

12. How would this responsibility impact on your other personal relationships? Will this cause resentment for time that must be devoted to being a caregiver?

What to Do and What to Avoid

If, after all your deliberations, you decide to assume responsibility for the person's medication care, remember these helpful tips.

1. Arrange for the two of you to meet with the person's doctor. When such a monumental change in responsibility is being proposed, it is important that members of the health care team be included. The doctor can give you valuable insight into the person's care and prognosis or expected outcome of his or her condition.

2. As an extension of point 1, have yourself listed as the *caregiver* on both the prescriber and pharmacy records.

3. Begin with less intrusive methods and progress to more hands-on involvement if you have to. Provide that which is actually needed! If a phone call twice a day to remind the person to take medication will get the desired results, then do this and only this.

4. Don't fix things that are working safely even though they may seem strange or ineffective to you. You will risk increasing confusion.

5. Don't get fancy. Simplify, simplify. If you are working with a person who has been having trouble remembering doses, refer to Chapter 18, Helpful Devices for Organizing Your Medications. There are many resources and devices available to jog the memory. Use them freely when appropriate. In addition, you can have the person's pharmacist look over his or her medication regimen and make suggestions about how it can be simplified. It may be possible to consolidate doses or suggest changes to the prescriber that will allow the person to get similar therapeutic results with medication that offers easier administration. Simple plans that can be understood by anyone can decrease the potential for confusion and error.

6. Base new systems for remembering to take medication on something familiar to the person like meals or bedtime. Ultimately, the plan has to work for the person for whom you are caring, not just you.

7. Once you've selected a plan, don't get too fond of it. Try it for a week or two then reevaluate it. You'll probably need to make modifications or even start over entirely. This is not failure, it's progress.

8. Don't get discouraged. Get help and moral support from the health care team.

9. Even when the person seems unable to participate in the care in any way, explain your actions and any changes to him or her. A confused person may not understand why you are involved and may need continued reassurance.

10. Repetition has been shown to be very effective in helping older people learn new things. It won't hurt for you to say something like, "Hello, I'm here again to help you take your medication" every time you show up if the person gives evidence that he or she doesn't remember why you have appeared.

11. Enlist the help of an occupational therapist (OT) to assess the living situation if you have questions about it. See if you can get a referral or call the local hospital or clinic for information on OTs. OTs are very skilled in determining what environmental factors may be contributing to problems. You'll find out if problems exist and if they can be fixed. If poor lighting in the kitchen is making the reading of medication labels difficult, you'll get a recommendation from an OT to change it. The OT will check to see if the person has any daily activities that can be tied to taking medication doses thus making it easier to remember them.

12. You will need to know about all the person's medications. This includes making a list that shows why medication is being given, the name and dose of the medication, and when it is administered. See Chapter 5 on patient learning systems and prepare the suggested medication information forms.

13. If you will be obtaining prescription refills for the person, synchronize these refills. Make it easy on yourself by taking all the prescription bottles to the person's pharmacy. Arrange for the pharmacist to fill them so they all run out on the same day. This will make monitoring compliance easier for you and the pharmacist. It will also cut down on your trips to the pharmacy.

Assuring the Person's Safety

Consider the safety of the person you are helping. Second only to small children, elderly people with confusion or memory problems now constitute the largest group of people suffering from accidental poisonings. Don't take any chances. If you have any doubts that the person doesn't understand the risks of unintentional consumption of medication, install a lock on a kitchen cabinet or drawer and store all medications there. At the same time, consider all other household chemicals as potential hazards. Store them safely in a different place.

Bill of Rights

It is a good idea to ask the local nursing home to send you a copy of their "Patient Bill of Rights." These documents have been developed in institutions to help staff and residents focus on maintaining dignity in the face of a loss of function. The items listed in these documents remind both caregivers and the people for whom they care of their rights and responsibilities in the relationship they share.

Taking Care of Yourself

For you to maintain the stamina and motivation to help the person with their medications, you must devote some attention to your own needs.

Plan Time Away for Yourself

Always plan for the possibility that you will not be there to help. Your system should be simple, clear, and organized. With the person's permission, get someone else's input on how easily understood his or her medication system is. It is a good idea to have another person trained and waiting in the wings to assume your duties if you are called away for any reason. Remember to take time off for yourself. This helps you maintain your perspective on being a caregiver and lets you keep up the other roles you hold in your community.

Your Personal Safeguards

The role of caregiver gives you access to many personal aspects of the person's life. Treat information about the person with respect and confidentiality. You will be best protected from any allegations of mismanagement if you keep good records. Start a file. Keep *all* receipts. Make a note of anything unusual you see. *Date the note.* Document any gift you are given and the circumstances in which this takes place. Try to get local businesses to establish charge accounts for your person so keeping records will be easier and clearer. Otherwise, use a special checking account to pay for all purchases. Make sure everything you do with regard to the person is ethically and morally right. When you are not sure, contact a relative of the person, a county social worker, the pharmacist, or the prescriber.

The person's therapy should not wear out the caregiver. You must protect yourself and your health in order to be able to help anyone else. Do not attempt physical tasks that you know or suspect may be harmful to you.

If the person whom you are helping has a contagious condition, find out from the health care team what measures you will need to take personally to safeguard your own health.

Be Your Own Advocate

The importance of this is illustrated by the following example.

A loyal customer appeared in the pharmacy. He looked frazzled. He has a few stable chronic health conditions. His wife, a diabetic with severe lung disease, had been diagnosed with a bone infection. She was started on home intravenous (IV) therapy. He was delighted she could be treated at home. While nurses were coming to their home every other day, he was responsible for administering IV doses around the clock. He was getting up an hour before each dose to get it out of the refrigerator and warm it up. He administered the dose through her catheter then he cleaned everything up for the next dose. At best, he was getting 3 hours of continuous rest at any one time.

Finally, he put his foot down. Things had to be made more simple or he just couldn't continue. Amazingly, within several days, the entire therapy had been adjusted and the situation was manageable for him. He reported it had been tough for him to "complain" when everyone was being so nice. He also said the worst thing about the ordeal was that he began to resent his wife, a woman to whom he had been married for 40 years.

An account of this incident is included here to highlight the fact that you as a caregiver must be your own advocate as well as an advocate for the other person. You should benefit by applying the principles and techniques found in this chapter. Be organized. Keep good records of the person's progress. Above all, remember that you are not alone. The entire health care team is there to support your work. Be comfortable asking for assistance.

Your Caregiver's Worksheet

When hospitals and nursing homes admit a person, they collect certain information about him or her. You and others who help you in your role as caregiver may need this same information. Medicaid numbers, insurance information of all kinds, and names and numbers for next of kin are just some of the things you might need to know. A sample worksheet is provided on the next page. Post the worksheet prominently on the refrigerator or on a wall near the telephone.

Caregiver's Worksheet

Todays date:

Your name, address, phone:

The person's name, address, phone:

(CIRCLE one)
This person:

speaks / writes / understands / English

speaks / writes / understands (another language)

Name of patient's physician, address, phone:

Pharmacy name & phone:

In an emergency call:

Next of Kin:

Insurance information:

Company   policy no.   telephone no.

Medicare information:

Advanced Directive (e.g. Living Will, Durable Power of Attorney for Health Care): YES NO

Where can it be found?

Diagnoses   *Name of Medicine*   *Strengths*   *Dosing Schedule*

Duties you are assuming as the caregiver (be specific):

Other caregivers and their duties as you understand them: includes Meals on Wheels, Visiting Nurse Service, cleaning service, and so on.

Name   Phone   Duties

(continued)

Medication-taking skills: (circle answer)

Can   Cannot   Open vials and bottles of medicine

Can   Cannot   Identify purpose of own medications

Can   Cannot   Remember to take medication on time

Can   Cannot   Administer own medication safely.

Can   Cannot   Be expected to take medication only as directed. Explain.

Can   Cannot   Obtain new and refill prescriptions from pharmacy without assistance. Explain.

Safety with medications or other hazardous substances is of concern. YES NO

Chapter 18

Helpful Devices
for Organizing
Your Medications

Numerous devices have been used to make medication compliance easier. This chapter lists some of the main types, their disadvantages, and their advantages.

Calendars

This is an uncomplicated solution to medication scheduling. Use one of your household calendars only for the purpose of keeping track of your medication. You can store it with your medication or hang it in the area in which you usually take your medications. Make a mark on the calendar each time you take a dose. At the end of each day, count the marks to make sure they equal the number of daily doses of medication that you take. If you are faithful to this method, you will avoid duplicate or missed doses. You can use a pocket calendar to keep track of doses when you are away from home.

Disadvantages of Calendars

This method does require some basic reading skills and the ability to learn and remember the goal of the system. In addition, it requires you to open and close your medication containers and to read and interpret the labels each time a dose is taken.

Advantages of Calendars

One particularly attractive aspect about this method is that the medication remains in its original packaging until it's time for you to take it. This assures you that it is properly labeled and has been under proper storage conditions up to the time you take it. Another good feature is that it is inexpensive and easily understood.

Daily Pill Boxes

Pill boxes are available as single compartment and multiple compartment containers. To use them, you remove an appropriate number of pills for one day's therapy from the original containers and place them in the box. The single daily box is designed to hold all the medications you take in one day. The multiple compartment container can hold either all your doses for several days or can be used to hold multiple doses for a single day as shown in the illustration on the next page.

These boxes are best if used for holding all the medications needed for one dosing time. The single com-

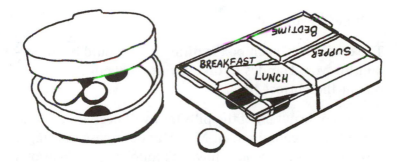

Single day medication boxes.

partment box is not as satisfactory if a number of medications must be taken at different times each day. If you have several daily dosing times and use single compartment boxes, you will need each pill box to be labeled with the time each dose should be taken. This is because you may be taking different medications at one dosing time than at another, for example, lunchtime as opposed to bedtime doses. Let me give you an example.

Mrs. Handes takes three different medications each day. We will call them A, B, and C. She has to take medication A three times a day, each morning, noon, and bedtime. She takes medication B twice a day, in the morning and at bedtime. At bedtime, she takes medication C. She is having trouble remembering which doses she has and hasn't taken. If Mrs. Handes wants to put her medications for each dose in individual boxes, her boxes would be labeled morning, noon, and bedtime. The medications would be distributed in the individual boxes like this:

morning: A and B

noon: A

bedtime: A, B, and C

The contents of each box is different. It would be important for Mrs. Handes to take the contents of the correct box at the correct time.

Some people put all of the pills they will need for a whole day into one container. In Mrs. Handes's case the single compartment box would have the following medications in it: A, A, A, B, B, and C.

Disadvantages of the Daily Pill Box

In this case, Mrs. Handes would just have a handful of unlabeled pills in her single compartment box. This means she'd have to distinguish between one medication and another based on its physical appearance. Since medications come in a variety of shapes, sizes, and colors that are routinely changed, there is potential for serious error.

One study showed that about 50 percent of elderly people tested could not consistently identify colors of tablets. With the diminished visual capacity of many elderly people, there is a significant risk of misidentification of medication when a person relies on color.

Advantages of the Daily Pill Box

Having to set up the box only once a day is likely to improve your chance of taking all your daily doses as directed. Any errors made in setting up the box would be perpetuated only for one day.

The 7-Day Pill Box

These boxes will accommodate 7 days worth of medication. Generally, they are a simple rectangle with seven compartments as illustrated on page 176. Some boxes will also allow you to separate multiple daily doses. These usually have seven rows and four columns of compartments where medicines can be stored. The box is

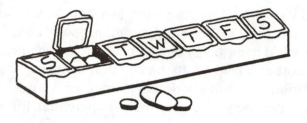

Simple 7-day (weekly) pill box.

marked with the days of the week and times of day such as morning, noon, evening, and bedtime as well as the days of the week as illustrated on page 177. For the right person, these are fine. The key is to identify whether you will be safe with the system.

Disadvantages of the 7-Day Pill Box

If you have already noted difficulties in learning and remembering new information, these pill boxes or "med minders" are probably a bad choice. The boxes may add just enough new information to really confuse you. Sometimes elaborate schemes like these 7-day pill boxes can lead to unintentional mismanagement of medications.

Some manual dexterity is needed to remove the desired pills without spilling the contents of the other compartments in the box.

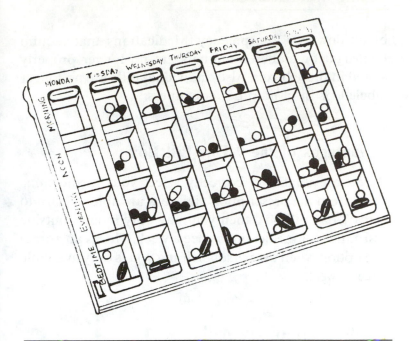

Weekly pill box for multiple daily doses.

You should be aware that whoever "sets up" the box with medications must do it accurately. Otherwise, there is the risk of giving incorrect medication *for a full week*. The person who administers the pills has to understand the system. The correct compartment for each dose has to be selected for each dosing time.

Storage conditions are not ideal in medication boxes. The United States Pharmacopoeia (USP) standards for the making, distributing and storing of medications are discussed in Chapter 19, Medication Storage and Disposal. Air and humidity can get in and cause drugs to break down or lose potency. Medications that require light-tight or amber containers are no longer properly stored in these boxes. Also, individual pills are no longer labeled or in child-proof containers.

Advantages of the 7-Day Pill Box

If you are unable to correctly select your medications doses from the prescription vials, but are able to learn to use a 7-day pill box, then you may only require outside assistance for medications once a week. This is an attractive option when the person helping you is only available once a week.

High Technology Aids

There are a wide array of alarm boxes, containers with timers, and boxes with caps that record the time the box was opened. These are "high tech" options whose usefulness only you can determine. An example is shown in the illustration on the next page.

Disadvantages of these Products

This group of products seem to require more skills than the others reviewed here. They frequently require programming and in-depth directions for use. Often, they have very small spots that must be pushed in order to set the various clocks and alarms. They seem a bit diminu-

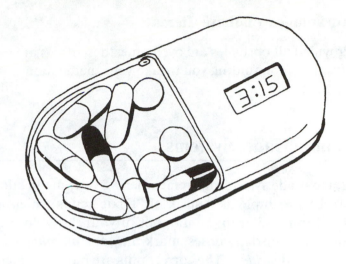

Pill box with alarm.

tive for elderly hands that may not have the dexterity of the inventor of the product.

Many of these items are sold through catalogs so you'd need to buy the item sight unseen. Before ordering, you need to find out if the company selling it has a return goods policy in case the product is not appropriate for you.

In products with an alarm, there is a possibility that you might not be able to hear the alarm when it rings because of its low volume and high pitch. Give it a try before you buy one or if you purchase through a catalog, verify the return policy first.

Advantages of these Items

Provided all obstacles are overcome, these items are very effective in reminding you to take your medication doses on time.

Home-Made Systems

Home-made systems for remembering your medications can be as simple as a stack of "Dixie" cups which are equal in number to the number of your daily doses. If you take four daily doses, mark the cups *morning, noon, supper,* and *bedtime.* The correct pills are put in each cup, and the cups are stacked on each other. When the morning dose is taken, that empty cup is moved to the bottom of the stack. This exposes the next dose to be taken. Similar systems have been devised with egg cartons. This type of system is appropriate only for daily use, not permanent storage. Some manufacturers have devised similar systems that allow you to store even liquid medications needed for the day. See the illustration on page 181.

Disadvantages of Home-Made Systems

The pills are exposed to improper storage conditions. Furthermore, because the pills would be open to view, this approach is risky for any small children who may find their way into your home. Safety can be improved by placing the stack of cups in a cupboard out of sight.

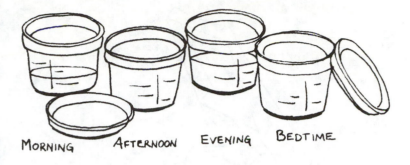

MORNING   AFTERNOON   EVENING   BEDTIME

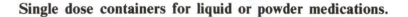

Single dose containers for liquid or powder medications.

Advantages of Home-Made Systems

Some of these systems are well known to elderly people and, thus, do not require learning a new method. These systems are simple and inexpensive.

Breaking Tablets

Occasionally, your doctor may direct you to take some fraction of a tablet. Special devices to safely split tablets are available from most pharmacies. Some alternatives are to cut the tablets with a razor blade or knife or to break them with your hands. Pharmacists can demonstrate how to break your particular tablets, and some pharmacists will routinely break the tablets for their patrons. An example of one popular device used for splitting tablets is shown in the illustration on page 182.

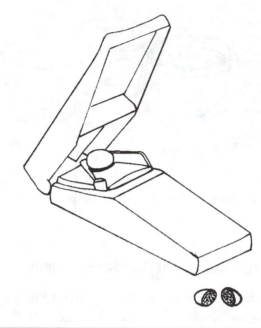

A popular style of tablet breaker.

Disadvantages of Tablet Splitting Approaches

The splitting device must be purchased. Knives and razor blades are more likely to shatter the tablet than the other methods. In addition, injury can easily be sustained with these makeshift devices. Popping the tablets apart with your hands can be difficult even without a physical disability. Decreased sensation in your hands, a common problem in the elderly, can eliminate breaking the tablets yourself as an alternative. Getting your pharmacist to break the tablets will mean you must give him or her advance warning that you will be needing the medication.

Advantages of Tablet Splitting Approaches

The pill splitter makes a clean break, is easy to operate, and is less likely than the other methods to cause you injury. The other methods are available in most homes and do not require a special purchase. Having the pharmacist demonstrate the breaking of your tablets is helpful since some tablets have special features that allow them to be more easily broken than others.

Crushing Tablets

There are several ways to crush tablets so you can recover the powder. Before crushing any tablet or capsule, consult your pharmacist to be sure the delivery of the correct dose will not be affected. Some products are formulated to release medication over a specific period of time. Crushing these products will result in improper dosing. One approach is to crush the tablet between two spoons. A mortar and pestle, found in many kitchens for crushing herbs, also works well for this purpose. A tablet crusher is available at many pharmacies.

Disadvantages of the Different Methods

It is more difficult to recover all the powder from the first two methods. This could lead to inaccurate dosing.

Advantages of the Different Methods

The first two methods have the advantage of no additional purchases being necessary. The crusher is easy to operate and contains the powder in a small jar. It is relatively inexpensive.

Conclusion

Devices and systems to guarantee that medications are taken as prescribed are readily available. It is extremely important to be sure the approach chosen makes sense to the person using it. The most familiar method is a good starting place.

Chapter 19

Medication Storage and Disposal

❖❖❖❖❖❖❖❖❖❖❖❖❖❖❖❖❖❖❖❖❖❖❖❖❖❖❖❖❖❖❖❖❖❖

This chapter focuses on the storage of medications. Proper storage of medication assures its safety and effectiveness. Improper storage can lead to medications that are less effective than they should be. Factors that affect the viability of your medications both in the pharmacy and in your home are discussed. There is information to help you choose an appropriate location to store your medications. The types of containers available are reviewed with the merits and drawbacks of each.

Protecting Medications from Breakdown

Medications are chemicals that are affected by the variables of storage. They break down faster in some environments than in others. Generally, the breakdown is not into a harmful substance, but into a chemical that is not as active as the original medication. The most critical factors influencing the chemical stability of medications are:

1. Temperature

2. Light

3. Humidity

4. Exposure to air

Temperature

Temperature can affect the stability and quality of medications. To maintain the potency of your medications you should know the temperature at which to store them.

Most tablets, capsules, and powders are stored at "controlled room temperature." This means that the refrigerator will be too cold and over the refrigerator will be too hot. Some medications, however, require refrigeration or freezing. The United States Pharmacopoeia (USP) publishes strict definitions of critical temperature conditions. These definitions are used by U.S. drug manufacturers and retailers to determine how medication will be stored.

Temperatures are defined in this way by the USP.

1. Cold: Any temperature less than 46°F (8°C). A refrigerator is a cold place in which the temperature is held between 36° and 46°F (2° to 8°C). A freezer is a cold place in which the temperature is held steady between 4° and -14°F (-20° and -10°C).

2. Cool: Any temperature between 46° and 59°F (8° and 15°C). An article for which storage in a cool place is directed may be stored in a refrigerator unless otherwise specified.

3. Controlled room temperature: Any temperature between 59° and 86°F (15° and 30°C). Most medications are stored at controlled room temperature. If the building that houses the medications is not temperature controlled, it may not meet these requirements in the cold of winter or heat of summer.

4. Warm: Any temperature between 86° and 104°F (30° and 40°C).

5. Excessive heat: Any temperature above 104°F (40°C).

When no specific storage requirements or limitations are provided, it is understood that the storage conditions include protection from moisture, freezing, and excessive heat.

Light

You have probably noticed that most medications are dispensed in amber-colored containers. A number of chemical reactions can be initiated in medications by exposure to light. To protect the medication from this breakdown, it should be stored both in the amber container and away from direct light.

Humidity

Moisture is a critical ingredient in many chemical reactions involving medications. High humidity can greatly hasten the rate at which medications become inactive. Some of the most humid places in your home are:

1. The refrigerator

2. The cabinets over your stove

3. Bathrooms with showers or tubs in them.

All these areas are too humid for the storage of medications. The traditional bathroom medicine cabinet needs a new name and function. It is actually a poor place to store medication because the humidity and heat fluctuate in and out of acceptable ranges.

Exposure to Air

The USP specifies that most medications be dispensed in tightly sealed containers. Exposure to air may speed evaporation of ingredients in medications or allow them to break down faster than they otherwise would. The classic example of problems in medication quality caused by exposure to air is the evaporation of the nitroglycerin from sublingual nitroglycerin tablets. Considerable testing was done to determine that this medication should be stored only in amber glass vials with a metal screw cap to seal the container tightly. Repackaging nitroglycerin tablets in any other type of container allows the active ingredient to evaporate.

Other Factors Affecting Medication Storage

Medication storage should be undertaken with the above suggestions. Other factors must also be considered. One is assuring accessibility of medications to the people who will administer or take them, while limiting access to people like children and adults with confusion or memory problems who might not be able to make rational decisions about medication consumption. The other concern is to maintain proper labeling on all medication containers. Prescription and OTC medications come packaged with labeling that identifies their name, use, and dose.

Currently, there is no nationally accepted policy on where to store medications. An informal survey of pharmacists reveals the following suggestions for medication storage in the original closed container. They meet the criteria established above.

1. Store in the cabinet where you store your canned goods, but not over the refrigerator or stove.

2. Store in your underwear drawer.

3. Store in a locked tackle box on the kitchen table.

When medication is transferred from its original container to a device that is intended to aid memory such as those described in Chapter 18, the storage conditions are rarely optimal. Few "med minder" boxes protect medication from light, air, or humidity. In addition, these boxes do not have safety closures. However, it is doubtful that quality is seriously compromised by storing medication in a daily pill box minder. The weekly kind of medication box presents a greater risk for drug breakdown and safety concerns. Certainly the repackaging of medications into unlabeled containers holding more than a week's worth of medication increases risks to people and medications.

Medication Containers

Container characteristics are also defined by the USP. They include that the container be clean prior to filling; that the container be made of material that will not interact with or alter the strength, quality, or purity of the contents and that it be light-resistant, well-closed, and tightly sealed.

The containers in which you purchase prescription and OTC medications meet the USP guidelines for package quality and safety. The memory aids and other containers you might use in repackaging medications generally do not meet these criteria. Neither do other makeshift medication containers like boxes, jars, drawers, and paper cups.

Disposal of Medications and Devices

Deciding to Dispose of Medication

Once a medication has been obtained, we have a tendency to want to keep it. Saving medications is not always a good idea, however. A few guidelines are possible for determining when to throw medication away.

Throw it away if:

1. The color, consistency, or smell has changed.

2. You've had the prescription bottle for six months or more.

3. You've had an open container of OTC medication for 6 months or more. This implies that you have noted on the container the date the product was opened.

4. The expiration date on the medication container is past.

5. You no longer are being treated with the medication.

If you've stored an unopened container of OTC medication under ideal conditions, you may keep it until one of the conditions above occurs.

How to Discard Medication

Discarding medication is usually as easy as emptying the contents of the bottles into the toilet and flushing. Cancer chemotherapy medications may have special disposal requirements. Ask your pharmacist or nurse for specific instructions.

Needles and Syringe Disposal

There is now a greater awareness of the dangers of some items used in injectable medication therapy. Because they are considered hazardous wastes, any items that contain body fluids like blood or pus must be disposed of in a special way. This includes the needles and syringes and any dressing material that has blood or pus on it. Safe disposal of these items is both important and easy.

Follow Local Regulations

Each state will have its own laws and regulations on this issue. Basically, these are designed to keep people from coming in contact with hazardous substances. In some states, needles and syringes must be disposed of in specially marked red "sharps" containers. The illustration on the next page depicts one such container designed for destruction of needles and syringes. The full container can only be collected by certain licensed disposal personnel.

Disposing of Hazardous Waste

Locate your local disposal business by looking in the yellow pages. The representative of this company has a

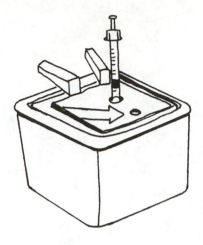

Needle/syringe destruction and disposal unit.

wealth of information and will be more than happy to talk with you about it. You may find that while the business also collects trash and recyclables, it has another mechanism for dealing with hazardous waste. Since not just any container meets the legal requirements, disposal businesses furnish the required type of container. The company representative picks up your specially marked and sealed containers when they are full. The containers are sent to a government approved incineration site and burned. When the waste has been properly destroyed, you receive a certificate stating that fact.

Proper storage and safe disposal of medications and associated devices protects you, other people, and your medication investment.

Chapter 20

Traveling with Your Medication

A change in your routine activities, such as traveling away from home, should not disrupt your medication therapy. To safely continue therapy, several issues need to be addressed. First, you'll need to decide what medication to take with you. Then you need to be sure that you will have access to your medications and that they will be stored under the best conditions. Finally, you will want to anticipate possible problems and emergencies and decide how to handle them should they occur.

What Should You Take With You

How much medication should you take? Calculate the number of days you will be gone. Multiply the number of days you'll need medication by the number of daily doses. To this number add 10 days to cover days before you leave and a couple of days following your return. This should allow you to you change your plans and not run into medication shortages. You can check your calculations by calling your pharmacist for help.

Access to Your Medication

Carry your medications with you in a secure bag that you'll be unlikely to lose. A medication box to hold the doses you need while traveling is handy. This way, you aren't flashing around big bottles of pills and giving airport or bus terminal undesirables the wrong ideas.

The fewer bags you are toting, the more likely you are to arrive with all of them. Never put your hand luggage down where you cannot watch it, and never let a stranger or new acquaintance watch your bags for you.

Proper Storage

Proper storage is generally not a problem if you have planned for the trip. Travel by car will allow you to put all your medication in a cooler with a couple of reusable freezer bags in it. Ice will work, but if it melts and leaks it could cause your medications to end up floating in water. The water can damage the medication as well as the labeling. Dry ice may make the medication too cold. Carry the cooler in the car with you. This will keep your medicine from becoming too warm in the trunk in the summer or too cold in the trunk in the winter.

Travel by bus, train, or airplane tends to restrict the number of items you can comfortably carry with you. Take your medication in a totebag with you onto the carrier. Don't ever check your medications with your luggage. The luggage compartments of trains or buses are not heated or, in the case of air travel, not always pressurized.

If you use a medication that requires refrigeration, you may find that a tiny portable cooler or one of the zipper travel bags made especially for insulin and its related equipment is helpful. An example is shown in the illustration on page 198. You can find these in pharmacies and mail-order health catalogues. Don't part with your medication or put it in the carrier's refrigerator. You may forget to retrieve it when you disembark.

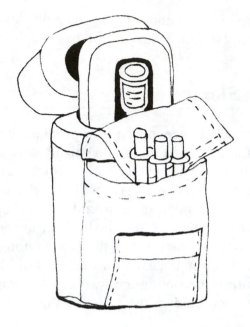

Travel pouch for diabetic supplies.

Handling a Crisis

Your medication diary can be a blessing in times of crisis when you and your medication are separated or if you are taken ill. It would contain all the information about your medication along with your doctor's name and phone number. Take it with you. Carry it in your hand luggage. Leave a list with a friend if you haven't memorized all your medication information. That way, if all your medication and lists are separated from you there will be a backup list.

If you lose your medications, try to contact your doctor or pharmacist to see if you can have the prescriptions called to a local pharmacy. If this fails, ask hotel personnel or your friends about a nearby physician. Make an immediate appointment. If this is not possible, you can always go to an "Urgent Care" facility or as last resort to an Emergency Room.

Don't try to tough it out without medication for the duration of your trip. You could have serious health consequences. Your trip will be less likely to upset your health if you are continuing your regular medication regimen.

Chapter 21

Addiction and Drug Dependence

In the course of taking medications, most people eventually stop and ask, "Is this medication addictive?" This chapter will introduce some of the terminology used when discussing drug addiction and physical dependence. It will explain how tolerance to medication effects differs from addiction and dependence. You will become acquainted with the basic concepts of physical dependence and drug addiction.

Better Health Through the Use of Medications

Be assured that most of the medications you take will not cause addiction or dependence. This is true even if you take them for a lifetime. The taking of medications chronically for legitimate medical conditions and with medical supervision is a health-seeking behavior. Discontinuing these medications could lead to the medical condition's being inadequately treated. However, it is unlikely that discontinuing them would cause any new physical discomfort as would occur with addiction or dependence.

With the use of medications on a daily basis, however, it is possible to develop a tolerance to some of the drug's effects. For example, if you are taking a medication that has drowsiness as a side effect, it is possible that you may develop a tolerance to the drowsiness without losing the beneficial effects from the medication. This does not mean you are addicted or dependent on the medication. Your body has simply adapted to some of the medication's effects. You can also develop tolerance to the beneficial effects of some medications, particularly narcotic pain medications like codeine or morphine. This means that to get the same effect you obtained when you first began taking the medication, you would have to take more of it.

Physical Dependence

Physical dependence refers to a physiological or body chemistry change that occurs because of the medication you are taking. The change in a person's body that occurs from taking the medication makes repeated use of the medication necessary. If the medication is not taken, the person may experience symptoms of withdrawal. For example, after months of regular consumption of some sleeping medications, a person can experience an unpleasant, even dangerous, physical reaction if the medication is not taken. It is as if the person's body is missing something without the medication.

The initial reason for taking the medication is for its therapeutic effects. A secondary reason for taking it is to keep from experiencing withdrawal from the medication.

Physical dependence can occur with *repeated* use of narcotics and some other medications. One of the facts the Food and Drug Administration (FDA) considers when it allows medications to be sold without prescription is their lack of ability to cause physical dependence.

Addiction

Addiction has to do with both the body and behavior of a person using a medication or drug. It means the person feels driven to find and use the medication or drug. This drive leads to what is called "drug seeking behavior." In part, the designation, addict, depends on what your society or culture sees as a problem. In the United States, society still tolerates physical dependence and addictive behavior related to tobacco, but it condemns physical dependence and addictive behavior of heroin use. Both are addictions, and both are harmful to the person.

Where physical dependence is established, the drug-seeking behavior is mainly what a society uses to determine whether it will tolerate the addiction. When the drug-seeking behavior involves harm to other people or property, a drug or medication is generally not allowed to be used without restriction in a society. Thus, heroin addiction is not tolerated, in part, because it involves crimes against members of society. Tobacco addiction harms mainly the person using it, but is not currently associated with serious harm to other people, so it is allowed in most societies. As information about harmful effects to other people becomes available about an addiction, for example damage to nonsmokers by "second-hand smoke", a society's tolerance of the addiction changes.

Tailoring Therapy to Individual Needs

While few of the medications you receive will cause physical dependence, this is an issue worth discussing with the members of your health care team. Our society avoids dependence on medications. There are times, however, that taking medication with a risk of dependence may be the best or only alternative available.

When Physical Dependence is the Only Alternative

There are times when developing dependence to a medication is considered the only alternative. In these cases, there should be:

1. An appropriate medical purpose such as the treatment of terminal cancer pain.

2. A therapy goal that takes into account the withdrawal syndrome should the medication be stopped. A commitment must be made to persons with a short life expectancy to continuously provide the dependency-causing medication without interruption so that withdrawal is avoided.

3. A stable supply of the medication is made available to the patient thus eliminating the need for him or her to engage in drug seeking behaviors such as lying, theft, or illegal purchases.

When Physical Dependence is a Problem

When people with no terminal disease suffer from chronic pain, the approach to pain relief is different. A 60-year-old person with painful arthritis can be expected to live 25 to 30 more years. To treat this person with medications such as narcotics that create physical dependence could cause many problems. Because of medication tolerance, it is unlikely that the narcotics would relieve the pain for long without the person having to increase the dose. Also, narcotics may affect a person's ability to function in his or her daily activities, so the quality of life is not enhanced. Finally, the person in this situation would undoubtedly meet many doctors who disagree with the concept of treatment with dependency causing medications. The outcome would be poor pain control and the need for the person to alter his or her behavior in a way that would help to secure the medications. Addiction is characterized by the development of these drug-seeking behaviors.

Drug-Seeking Behavior

With the development of a physical dependence, addictive drug-seeking behaviors can be established. Addiction violates all the ideas health professionals have about human dignity. It puts people in a situation where they may violate their moral and ethical standards to avoid withdrawal from the medication on which they are physically dependent. These are some of the reasons addicting medications are avoided by prescribers. Therefore, every attempt is made to provide rehabilitative therapy and medications that will allow each person to live a normal life.

Many people will experience drug seeking behavior personally or with friends or family members. Perhaps as a result of an injury or fall, a prescription for a mild narcotic will be given. If the pain does not go away completely, the prescription may be refilled. As time goes on the refills run out, and the doctor must be consulted about the narcotic. If the person is at the point of drug-seeking behavior, he or she may dramatically describe the pain and try to get another refill. This creates a difficult situation. It is best if the entire health care team and family are involved. They can work together to withdraw the offending medication and free the person from the addiction.

This chapter has only introduced you to the terminology and concept of medication dependence and addiction. Contact your area Alcohol and Other Drug Abuse Counselor for confidential advice. Don't let a situation become a problem. Get help.

References

American Medical Association White Paper on Elderly Health: Report of the Council on Scientific Affairs. (1990). *Archives of Internal Medicine, 150,* 2459–2472.

Col, N., Fanale, J. E., Kronholm, P. (1990). The role of medication noncompliance and adverse drug reactions in hospitalizations of the elderly. *Archives of Internal Medicine, 150,* 841–845.

U.S. Senate Special Committee on Aging. (1988). *Developments in Aging, (1)*2. Washington, DC.

Kaestle, C. F., Damon-Moore, H. (1991). *Literacy in the United States* (pp 98–99). New Haven, CT: Yale University Press.

Kosnik, W., Winslow, L., Kline, D., Rasinski, K., Sekuler, R. (1988). Visual changes in daily life throughout adulthood. *Journal of Gerontology: Psychological Sciences, 43*(3), 63–70.

Index

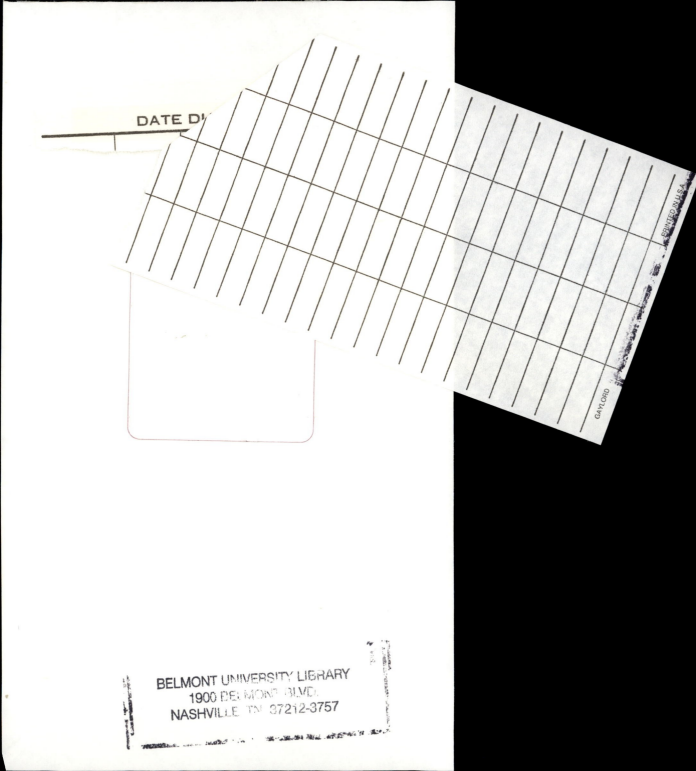

DATE D